Bladder Cancer Stories

littleoldladywho

Publishing Data

First published 2021 Sliding Scale Books (LOLWPB02)

Plaza De Andalucía 1, Campofrío, 21668, Huelva, Spain.

(c) Copyright Littleoldladywho 2021

Design by Frank Fisher

ISBN 978-8412202960

All rights reserved.

The right of Littleoldladywho to be identified as the author of this work has been asserted in accordance with the Copyright Designs and Patents Act 1988, sections 77 & 78.

No part of this publication may be reproduced, stored in a retrieval system or transmitted in any form or by any means without the prior permission of the publisher and author or her agents.

The publishers and author can accept no legal responsibility for any consequences from the application of information instructions or advice given in this publication.

To those who care with empathy and dedication.

Contents

Bladder Cancer Stories	9
A 'long-tail' life	10
My year of eating Cheetos (2015)	11
Quick symptoms-to-diagnosis roundup	12
Waking in the night	14
First symptoms	15
The UTI Group	15
Conversations with UTI Group Admin	16
Telling my children	19
Scan - 5th Sept 2016	20
The womb exploratory operation	21
Uroscopy - Oct 2016	22
It's cancer	22
Mama's cancer	23
How long is time under a green sheet?	23
First TURBT - Nov 2016	24
The lazy nurse and the angel	25
Full 70s?	26
Results	27
Fight Bladder Cancer group (28 Nov 2016)	28
CT Scan - (5th Dec 2016)	28
CT scan side effects (FBC group 6 Dec)	29
Results (FBC Group Nov 2016)	29
Acceptance - Dec 2016	30
Go home and enjoy Xmas!	31
Fears (FBC group 23 Dec 2016)	32
Writing my Memoir	33

Workplace exposure (FBC group 29 Dec 2016)	33
What causes cancer?	34
Night fears (FBC group 1 Jan 2017)	35
Second TURBT (FBC group 10 Jan 2017)	36
Calls of nature	36
Male nurses (in Spain)	37
Decision time	41
Lymph nodes (FBC group)	42
Feeling 'Waspish' (FBC Group 9 jan 2017)	42
Pre-ops for Radical Cystectomy (30 Jan)	43
Pre op nerves (FBC group 31 Jan)	44
The first days after the operation	44
On the ward	47
Healing	48
'Blanda Facil' - Feb 2017	49
Kidney pain	50
A rebel without a coffee	51
Abdominal support - Feb 2017	52
Home! ... Not home	52
Wafer changes, leaks etc.	53
Do I smell?	53
Unbroken nights! (FBC Group Feb 2017)	54
Telling the world (on my Facebook page)	55
Night Sweats (FBC group)	56
Bicarb' (FBC group 4 March)	56
Neighbours' empathy	57
Oncology and chemotherapy	57
Tiredness (FBC group 11 March)	58
The Day Hospital	59

Chemo side effects (FBC group 17 Mar)	59
My 60th Birthday April 2017	60
Travel with a stoma	61
3rd Chemo cycle	62
Thoughts on Chemotherapy	62
Housework!	63
Emotionally battered	64
A sneaky wee (June 2017)	64
A brush with 'Natural Medicine'	65
The Flamenco dress	66
Throat Problems	66
Blood spot (FBC group)	67
Sniffer Dogs?	67
Bag or bucket (FBC group)	67
Happy Christmas! (FBC group)	68
Extension tubes (FBC group)	68
Close the plug! (FBC Group)	69
Phantom bladder (FBC Group)	70
Stomaversary (FBC group 31 Jan 2018)	70
Missed Scan - FBC group	70
All clear - FBC group	70
'Transference'	71
Walking	72
Mother's day thoughts - FBC group	72
Data	73
Dramatic failure	73
Nutritional medicine (FBC group Nov 2018)	74
Leaks - FBC group	74
Gender confusion!	75

Toilets	76
Itchy skin (FBC group July 2019)	77
Self worth (FBC group June 2019)	77
Exercise	78
Another year (FBC 31 Dec 2019)	78
Zen and the art of ignoring sh** (2020, 3 years cancer Free)	79
Out walking	80
Diuretic - 15 Aug 2020	80
Swimming 'fun' - July 2021	81
Sex and relationships	82
You are not powerless	84
The End	85
Appendix	87
Thanks and acknowledgements	89

8

Bladder Cancer Stories

First word: If you have blood in your urine (outside of a monthly period) along with bladder irritation, don't take time to read this book yet. Get yourself to the doctor and ask for a cytology test. Hopefully, it's cystitis, or a very bad bladder infection, but in any case that is serious and needs sorting out. bladder cancer is treatable but it can be aggressive. Don't leave it too long to get checked out … I should know: I was very nearly too late! If you find blood in your urine when you go to the toilet, rather than blood that appears at other times, don't be stoical. Run, don't walk to your doctor, ask to be referred immediately to an urologist and ask for a cystoscopy.

Now that's done, here are my disclaimers.
This is not a guidebook. Because my diagnosis was so late this book covers the almost-worst-case scenario of very late stage but non metastasized bladder cancer. Because of that it may not cover your treatment for earlier stages. I hope it will give you hope that all may not be lost if your cancer returns.

At the time of writing I've been almost 5 years cancer-free and so, for me, this book is a bit of a celebration.

I'm opinionated: sometimes very opinionated. My writings here include rants on subjects that may not have been fully scientifically proven. I don't want you to take any of my comments as gospel, just as information and occasional humour. The sort of stuff people like me think of at times like this. It's written in diary format but many entries come from my posts on the Fight bladder cancer Facebook group. For privacy I haven't included any actual replies. Some earlier ones come from a cystitis support group on Facebook. I am forever grateful to both of these groups. There will be some comments on sex and 'girly-bits', so buckle up if you are easily offended.

So, here are my stories about my search for answers, my musings and some bits of info about some of the funny, and not so funny things that happened on my journey, and the mostly wonderful treatment I received. I also chat about what I did to support my chances of recovery.

A 'long-tail' life

We're all going to die. That's for sure. If it were possible to crack this fundamental certainty, I'm pretty sure Steve Jobs would have found it. As a lifelong 'lefty' it's pretty reassuring to me that the mega rich will suffer the same fate as I will in the end. Like almost everyone else, I'm dedicated to holding that day off for as long as possible: and I do dedicate myself to it! I'm having way too much fun to leave now.

How then, do I intend to help myself ensure the longest and healthiest and happiest life from now on?

For a start I needed to reverse the really bad habits I'd got into over the preceding few years. I believe that all these contributed in some small way to my system being overloaded. For those whose cancer has come completely out of the blue, I don't want to suggest that you in any way contributed to your illness. In my case I really believe that I did. That belief whether true or not did give me the feeling that if I'd put those things in, I could have some power to take them back out. It doesn't matter whether that's true or whether anyone believes that there's any scientific basis in these beliefs. Some people pray to their gods for a good outcome ... I was prepared to make changes.

Our whole digestive and excretory system is incredibly important to our general health. More important still, when those systems are under strain. This was what I'd failed to take any account of in my life. Altering my lifestyle in several ways was the least I could do to honour the surgeons' hard work, to honour my own incredible body, and to give myself as extended a life as possible.

I believe that in my case I'd let myself get out of hand in several ways.

I didn't drink enough water. I really wasn't fond of water and so I drank several cups of tea a day. When I was busy I forgot even that. Drinking enough helps the elimination process. While we're on elimination - I didn't get enough exercise. Added to that I sat in the same place all day making crafts and only getting up to go to the loo, and even then not often enough. As I said, I didn't drink enough.

Exercise helps your body to move the fluids through the lymphatic system. The lymphatic system is our body's 'sewerage system', collecting and removing all the waste that passes out of our blood vessels from immune responses. So that's why you get raised glands in your neck if you have a throat infection. Those lymphatic glands are overworking at that time.

I was also overweight. About 20-25 kilos overweight. This is common in people who don't drink enough water. Maybe we mistake thirst for hunger? I'd been living on a poor and lazy diet, high in sugars, especially fructose, high in preserved meats and high in foods to which I had an allergy or at least an intolerance to (this was all proved in allergy testing a year later).

And ... I had undiagnosed depression.

My year of eating Cheetos (2015)

Looking back it's obvious to me that all those poor choices were a symptom of depression. It's just that depression is not as obvious in sunny Andalusia. Every day I had at least one pack of Cheetos. More often than not, two. Well, they were cheap and they were 'carbylicious!' They weren't the only unusual thing I ate too much of that year. I'd also found tasty tasty pork scratchings in Lidl. The sort you used to get in England. Greasy, salty and crunchy. They used to give me diarrhoea because I ate too many of those as well. I was drinking at least six cups of decaffeinated tea a day. My working days were sedentary and only punctuated by getting up to go for a wee, a tea and the Cheetos. It was not a healthy way to live. I wasn't thinking of health. I was too busy concentrating on trying to dig us back out of the mess we'd been in financially the years before. As long as I kept doing the teaching and filled in the shortfall in the crafts income by working until midnight, It just seemed like I was doing my best, but we weren't getting far enough fast enough given that I owed money to family. I think my husband was depressed too. He was starting to spend more and more time on Facebook, joining groups who chatted about nothing in particular, or to be specific they deliberately talked of nothing challenging. I think it was a refuge from real life for him. I did start to resent how much time he was spending cut-off from the reality of our situation, while to my mind, I was shouldering the burden. This, of course, wasn't really fair because my husband was always on hand whenever there was a job within his capabilities, and whenever I asked him to do it. The problem was ... I didn't ask. I was more cut off than I realised. He would spend his days in his office, partly dealing with orders, and partly struggling with old equipment which barely functioned and also producing my books and YouTube videos. Whilst struggling with his own feelings of helplessness, my occasional bouts of stress-induced bad temper can't have helped.

Quick symptoms-to-diagnosis roundup

For people who are on the beginning of the road, I thought I'd give a very quick roundup of how I got to the stage of diagnosis, which took too long, at almost a year. I first noticed blood in my wee in early 2016. For about a year before that my urine had been smelling different. It actually wasn't an awful smell. I described it at the time as the smell of chicken soup, sweet and salty I suppose. I even went online with the question "What makes your urine smell like chicken soup?" There weren't any clear results from that search, although I wasn't the only one who was asking!

I went to the doc and got an appointment for a scan of my womb. The scan seemed to show there might be a polyp. I suddenly realised the blood in the toilet was from my urine and not gynaecological. There were some delays because I was on the list for a gynaecological operation for what they thought might be a polyp in my womb. Until that was done, they didn't seem interested in looking further. The night before that little operation my blood pressure went up (possibly anxiety) and my urine was deep burgundy red with blood. Nevertheless, in spite of the bleeding, they took me in and did the op', and found ... precisely nothing. It wasn't really surprising that this was a red herring as I'd had a previous cone biopsy for suspicious cells, so they felt that a problem in the womb was likely. After that I had to wait all of August because Spain effectively closes during that period.

In September I had a cystoscopy where they looked in my bladder with a camera. In October I had my first TURBT(Transurethral Resection of Bladder Tumour) in November, I then had a CAT scan and then I got the news I knew I would get. Initially my tumour was considered to be non-muscle-invasive but was aggressive, But the TURBT seemed to show that it might be muscle-invasive. There was some question as to whether an RC - Radical Cystectomy, in other words complete removal of the bladder, would be the way to go. So, another wait for Spanish Xmas before I had my second TURBT in January and straight away was scheduled for an RC. I was delighted by then to be given this chance because by that time I knew it was borderline. It was deep muscle-invasive and there was some effect on the lymph nodes. In February I had My Radical Cystectomy. I wasn't so scared because it was either that, or a terminal diagnosis.

Because this was a chance of life, I embraced my stoma and my bag and embraced the idea of Chemotherapy. Chemo was horrible. Truly horrible, but it was a 'belt and braces' job to make sure that no cancer cells lived to fight another day. I've started working again. Started swimming. Lost more than 20 Kilos (mostly deliberately). With hard work we've got over some financial and psychological problems, which were in many ways linked. I'm getting there. I'm telling this story because I was looking for this kind of info when it happened to me. What might happen and when. I was pretty scared and I was at first horrified at the thought of a stoma. That changed pretty quickly.

If you've recently been diagnosed, or even if you just think you might have BC, keep pushing the timetable particularly for that first cystoscopy. Then It's a rollercoaster. You just have to buckle up. Don't be afraid, because fear doesn't help. Do your research, or ignore it, whichever will make you feel most comfortable. I found knowledge reduced my fear.

The Fight bladder cancer Facebook group really helped. Whenever I felt lost I asked for directions. Not everyone agrees but that doesn't matter. I mean it *really* doesn't matter what other people think of your choices. That's the one thing I definitely learned. It's your disease. From all the available advice and support, you take the bits you need.

So let's go back to early 2016. Here's the story in full through ranting and rambling, discussions with people online, with family and friends, and messages on the facebook groups. These will usually be marked FBC group (Fight bladder cancer): I've left these as rambling discussions to show the nature of the process of trying to find out what the heck is wrong with you.

Waking in the night

I'm sure it's common to all of us with bladder problems, that we wake in the night, often several times with the need to go to the toilet. Then possibly only an annoyingly small trickle when we do. The worst part of this though is the staying awake and all the 4 am what-ifs.

This is a scary time. We often beat ourselves up because we tell ourselves we're being stupid and we imagine other people are thinking that we're hypochondriacs, and to be fair they often do. Several times on a cystitis page on Facebook, I read about people having confusing symptoms, and I know my symptoms confused me and I kept flip-flopping from the certainty that I had bladder cancer, to the hope that it was something lesser. One thing which didn't help as much as people meant to was the kindly but ill informed "It's probably nothing."

First symptoms

I did have bad cystitis about 2 decades ago followed by occasional bladder discomfort throughout the years. Occasionally in the decade before my diagnosis I'd treated this with an antibiotic available over the counter here in Spain. I seemed to have worse problems when travelling or when I was stressed. The discomfort was usually mild however and usually went away on its own. On one trip to Denmark in 2015 I thought I'd seen a little blood in my wee, but then contented myself that it was because I'd just eaten a salad containing beetroot. Almost exactly a year later the blood reappeared.

The UTI Group

When my symptoms were getting worse, and I started to feel there was something wrong. I started looking on an UTI (Urinary Tract Infection) Group and I had several long conversations with the admin of this group, who suggested I try a particular 'protocol' to rid myself of any UTIs (Urinary Tract Infections). The longer I was in the group however, the more my symptoms, more specifically my test strip readings, looked different from theirs. Even though I didn't always agree with some of the weirder treatment options, this group possibly saved my life, partly by suggesting that I buy the urine test strips. As soon as I started testing and following my own version of the 'protocol' advised in the group, I realised I didn't have any obvious infection most of the time when I was experiencing discomfort. I had leukocytes but no nitrites whereas those who had infections usually had both, or just nitrites. I started to find granules in my urine. So, I started looking into stones and asked my doctor about this. He sent me for a radiology exam ... Nothing at all was seen in the X-ray!

Conversations with UTI Group Admin

Me: Hi R. I just joined the group. I found you by following some of your answers on a forum somewhere in the early hours of yesterday morning. I was just writing a piece outlining my recent problems *(I always write when I'm anxious about something.)*
Thanks for adding me. I have always been a fan of nutritional medicine since I cured myself of panic attacks largely by changing my diet. I'm under investigation by our local hospital for a polyp in the womb found when looking for the cause of what may have been bleeding from the womb or may have been an earlier UTI, or could even be bladder cancer. *(This was the first time I'd voiced my concerns about the possibility of cancer.)* I believe during the procedure of trying to get into the neck of my womb I was possibly infected with an antibiotic resistant UTI. Things are grinding slowly here because it's August in Spain. Yes, we are lucky there is a healthcare system but it's not perfect. I have been bleeding daily for getting on towards two months now and during this time have so far had three courses of antibiotics, none of which seem to have removed this aggressive infection. I have during this time tried making a lemon and ginger barley water which has had some but not complete success in relieving the symptoms. I'm a sceptic, but probably more sceptical about wonder drugs than about solid fact based nutritional medicines!

Me: Hi R. I'm living hand-to-mouth at the moment (very long story) so, rather than taking the pre-packed herbal supplements you recommend I'm going to try to make up a paste of stoned fresh olives, garlic, ginger and turmeric. It will taste bloody awful. I'm courageous if nothing else.

R: The active ingredient is oleuropein: you need the highest percentage you can find.

Me: It's very high in fresh uncured olive fruit.

R: Alright, it's highest in 'young olives' ... By which I presume it means unripened.

Me: Exactly as they are on my tree at the moment.

R: If you can get it down and keep it down, that would be awesome! And what a story it would make!!!

Me: I can let you know how it goes. I'll gather a bucketful and put them in my freezer. BTW Have you ever heard of this
R: ?
https://en.wikipedia.org/wiki/Lepidium_latifolium

(Lepidium latifolium, known by several common names including broadleaved pepperweed, pepperwort, or peppergrass, dittander, dittany, and tall whitetop, is a perennial plant that is a member of the mustard and cabbage family.)

I bought some from a herb seller here. I have had small calcium stones in my wee which appear whenever the inflammation level drops. This seems to help flush it as I hadn't seen any for weeks, then, after taking this they started coming out in my wee again.

Apparently these calcium deposits can form and hang around areas where there is damage and inflammation. Presumably they can hold on to infection too. Can be a sign of cancer of the bladder. But which comes first: Repetitive inflammation or cancer? Whether I have or haven't got this. I still need to clean up!

Whether it was the homemade cayenne/olive/garlic mix which I settled on, or the Lepidium Latifolium or just a coincidence I'll never know for sure, but whatever I was doing seemed to provoke my bladder to shed its 'hangers-on'. HOWEVER Before you go trying any of these weird mixes you should know that the mix of turmeric and garlic in large quantities also probably acted as a blood thinner. This may have caused some of the heavy bleeding described later. This story is just for interest and in NO WAY a recommendation. Consult your doctor if you have any of the symptoms mentioned in these pages.

Me: Hi R. I had tried insisting that they check me for cancer when I went to the emergency department with the bleeding,

I don't think they took me seriously . It was a small hospital and I guess if they saw two or three bladder cancers a year in Urology that would be a lot. Accident and emergency didn't seem to connect those dots. I had a 'radiografia'. Which I think was an X-ray, to see if I had stones or calcifications. They said I didn't, but I could feel grit in my wee. Where was that coming from? They said I needed to see an Urologist and I took it at the time that they were referring me.

When I mentioned this on the Cystitis group, someone said that some types of stones are radiotranslucent. Meaning they can't be seen on radiography. My radiography looked clear which is another reason why they weren't taking me seriously.

I wrote down a history of my symptoms. I was 'pissed off' and very worried by this time, so I went directly into the urology department, to find out why I hadn't yet got an appointment. Apparently, and shockingly, I wasn't on the list and should have gone back to my own doctor after the trip to the emergency room, to be referred. Something had been lost in translation, and I'd wasted nearly 2 months!

> **ME:** Hi R. Well, I'm not posting this on the FB page because it's a bit gross, but to add to the sum of your knowledge which I know is already impressive. Just now I passed a 'thing' which looks like it's been attached to the wall of my bladder, so some kind of damage which has been encrusted with calcium or uric acid deposits. It's kind of folded up but looks like it has been the size of a dime (I had to look your coins up). I knew something big was moving as it was very painful. I got some mosquito net and peed through it and that's how I caught it. I photographed and then double vacuum bagged and froze it. Now at least I have something to take to the doctor. Or I might even go directly to the hospital and insist they check it for cancerous cells. I've waited far too long already for them to dick-around without even bothering to check that out. Hoping it's nothing like that of course, but I have too many predisposing factors not to want to know.

(It) Looks like in some way the meds may be working even if just to put my bladder into enough shock to shrug off this thing.

I took photographs of what I now believe to have been a tumour, plus a note translated to the best of my ability into the hospital, and looked for someone who would take me seriously. Eventually I spoke to some important lady who I think was a kind of hospital administrator. It seems I was supposed to ask my doctor for an appointment after my emergency visit. I had assumed that having been in the emergency room that I would have been referred on to a specialist as a matter of course! I had wasted nearly 2 months! At least she took me seriously and made my appointment then and there.

Telling my children

I have to say here I'm not a big fan of keeping things from your family. I think talking is almost always good even if it feels bad at the time. Those people I know who have lost relatives to various cancers and who got through it the best, were always those who talked to each other all the way through.

I used the history of doctors visits etc. to tell my daughter that I thought there was a possibility that I had cancer. I didn't want to tell my eldest son, at least not yet. I didn't feel there was anything to be gained by it. He was going through a scare with his wife needing a mammogram. They had had a very tough couple of years of unhappy experiences with a loss followed by a birth and now their own cancer scare. They really had enough to worry about. At the time, emotionally I just wanted to swap me for her. Well of course that wasn't really a bargain to be had, and anyway I didn't want to die either. Her mammogram was clear: thank goodness. Clearly there are times when the decision has to be not to complicate other people's lives unnecessarily.

I wanted to tell my daughter first. She was very supportive in a really gentle non-freaked out way, which I was grateful for.

I just gave her the history so far of my visits to doctors and all the possibilities. I wanted her to be prepared if it turned out that it was cancer.

There's one more thing I remembered to tell my daughter which I'd forgotten until that time.

> **Me:** Last time I had a blood test ... maybe 9 months ago there was a high indicator on one component which the doc said could be a cancer indicator but could also just be because of an infection. Ahh yes I said, I was suffering from a bladder infection when they took the sample. Doh!
>
> **K:** Ahh I see. So it seems there are a few indicators. I can imagine why that might worry you in the early hours. Have you spoken to Frank about all of it? Still, there's a very good possibility that it will be nothing or something very minor, so don't start panicking and filling your head with what-ifs at this stage.
>
> **Me:** Yes, Frank knows. But there's nothing like talking to another girl!

Within a week or two, I had also told the rest of the family.

Scan - 5th Sept 2016

I got an appointment for a scan a month later. The scan showed a cloudiness. This first Urologist said he had an idea what the problem was and that I didn't need any more antibiotics. When he said this, I didn't read the right thing between the lines and I thought the shape of the cloud on my scan looked like a type of stone called Jackstones.

When I went for the uroscopy with a different urologist, it was delayed for a couple of hours while the antibiotics I needed to take took effect. I needed a strong set of antibiotics after that too. Absolutely convinced I got a hospital bug from the session in the gynae outpatients the month before. A horrible appointment where the patient who went in before me was not a 'live patient.'

She arrived in a specially covered blue tent. I had to wait until the room was mopped down afterwards too. A very disquieting experience that I really wanted to run away from. They still couldn't get into my womb and so they put me on the list for an operation under local anaesthesia.

> **Me**: Dear R, I had an appointment with an Urologist this morning. The scan did show 'something'. So it may be that UTIs are just a side effect of something more suspicious in my case. He told me to forget about UTIs and that he has another theory which he needs to check out with cytology. No more antibiotics for the moment, the cytology appointment is 3 weeks from now. I'm staying on the natural meds for now anyway and bah to his assertion that eating olives in their natural state will contribute to weight gain! (I am fat, though). The way I see it, the garlic/olives/cayenne mix, and the urinary tract tea seems to work for me. Although I hate taking it, it's a food albeit a nasty bitter one. I think it can't do any harm. The way I see if it's worth a try to shrug any more nasty things off my bladder in the 3 weeks I'm waiting for Cytology.

Uroscopy and biopsy - that is to say a look into the bladder with a camera and taking a little piece of tissue for testing.

The womb exploratory operation

The day before the operation I suddenly started bleeding more. I think it might have been high blood pressure from the stress so there was another overnight visit to Accident and Emergency. Then, that same day I had the gynae 'op. ' The results of which were clear. After this, they told me yes, I did have an infection which showed nitrites for which I was given antibiotics. This takes us up to early September or thereabouts. By this time I was convinced I had bladder cancer but I was still being treated like someone who Googled too much.

Uroscopy - Oct 2016

Uroscopy yesterday. My goodness I'd followed the advice to have a full bladder. It was painfully full. Why was the Urologist showing me a video of plastic bags blowing in the wind around a rubbish tip, I thought ... Oh no! That was the inside of my bladder! Very nice new urologist but not really the best news. I do have stones, but they are more encrustations on whatever else is hanging around on my bladder wall. The pressure at the end of my exam was so very great that I begged to be able to release it and the doctor just pulled out a kind of tray under me and left me to let go. Embarrassingly the flow seemed to last about 5 minutes but it was probably nearer 30 seconds. It was the weirdest feeling and something I would never normally do. I think the relief was not only from the release of bladder pressure but that finally I was on the road to being taken seriously. They took a biopsy, and I've been asked to come back tomorrow for the preliminary results.

Obviously there's a pretty strong chance that there is some kind of cancerous element to this, which I also thought because of the predisposing factor of having been exposed to large quantities of phthalates and pigments in the past in my work, but because I was being very proactive by this time I often came across the attitude that maybe I was using Google too much! And Doctors don't really seem to understand that exposure to chemicals through the hands of a busy craftswoman is really exposure. (I live in a mining area where only 'real men' get 'real' chemical exposure!)

It's cancer

I went back to urology the day after my uroscopy when 'Mr Burns' (that's who he looked like) told me that all bladder cancers were malignant. It wasn't easy translating machine gun Spanish, but that, I got. It was cancer. Mr Burns started to explain to me that my smoking for 10 years, 30 years ago was the probable cause.

Oh OK, (In my opinion) not the only cause, but more likely a contributory factor among many.

I go in next week for removal. They'll check and tell me the results. I've already been told bladder cancers are always considered malignant and so couldn't just be ignored, but that the stage is important. If it's not too deep, 'easy-peasy.' Whip them off and look for more in a year, then every 5 years. If they've gone through the bladder wall into deep tissue, well that gets serious. I'm really upbeat about it at the moment because finally I can let go and let them get on with it.

Since these things can be time-sensitive I'd like to have got to this point earlier, though!

Mama's cancer

One of the things which helped me enormously was my Spanish friend who I call Mama, going through cancer herself. She was going through it with a really positive, but also accepting attitude. She seemed very quickly to get through all the grief stages (which I never saw) to "It is what it is." Apparently it's really common for people to ask "Why me" but I never saw that in Mama. I was already concerned that I might have cancer myself as Mama was going through her treatment and her attitude really supported me. I thought, "I want to be like that" and so I was. So even though I had the same 4 am fears as everyone else, especially pre-diagnosis. There was a certain relaxation that diagnosis itself gave me. "See I was right." Now I can get on with looking at how much future I have and if there's any chance I can lengthen that. I found a book called Anticancer and I read it cover to cover.

How long is time under a green sheet?

Before my big operation which my sister (a theatre nurse) called my 'horrendoplasty', I had three smaller ops so one thing which I was getting used to was the relaxant. Maybe I became too used to it? Before the operation you are given a pre-op. Some kind of tranquiliser, probably morphine based. I'm sure it's a very important part of the process. I will forever call it 'no f***s juice', because that's exactly what it does for you. Oh yes, the spinal injection kills your lower body sensation and of course that's the most important part. The pre-op is what makes the local possible, because you really don't care from then on. Imagine the theatre always filled with twittery patients screaming out loud from fear rather than actual discomfort. Nobody needs that while they're working. With the pre-op there is no fear and strangely also, no sense of time. My first investigative operation on the womb took what felt like seconds and probably was only minutes. I'd only been given a proper 'op only because of previous issues which presented 'access difficulties'. My first TURBT (removal of tumour for biopsy - Trans Urethral Resection of Bladder Tumour) took a couple of hours waiting in the corridor and very little time actually in surgery. How much of a sense of time do I have? None. It was all almost instant. During my last very complicated TURBT when there was no waiting in the corridor and the actual operation took about two hours. It felt like 20 minutes. I was actually aware of some time passing on that one, so I did wonder if I was becoming too accustomed to the medication and starting to 'give one'.

First TURBT - Nov 2016

They took out a 5cm polyp/tumour and some other bits and bobs. Basically, they cleared out the junkyard. Of course that was never going to be the end of it. That was really just exploratory. Still I was pleased to have got to this stage.

My middle son and his girlfriend came to visit during this time. My son had made me laugh. He said, "do you want me to come over?" I jumped at the chance but asked if he could get the time off. He said "If I use the C word ... that usually works". He paused before the punchline ... "Give me time off C**t!" I was in hysterics. I don't usually use 'that word' and neither does he, but he, like his granddad (my dad) is never one to let a linguistic joke go undeveloped.

I was really grateful for this visit because it meant my husband could still go to a fair that we'd promised to attend. Since we were already pretty much penniless by this time, this was an absolute must too. I really didn't want to be on my own. It wasn't so much the being alone I minded. It was being relatively alone. Spanish patients always have at least one relative accompanying them at all times! I already found the sympathetic noises and looks a bit burdensome when they noted that I was alone between visits. Even though I was previously fine, I found myself being tearful when people were sympathetic.

I understand in the UK you go home straight after a TURBT. Here in Spain, I stayed for 5 days each time. I'm not sure if that is standard here or if I was a special case. I had irrigation for the first 24 hours. That is to say my bladder was washed with saline after the operation. Then they kept me in to recover. I think I lost quite a bit of blood though, especially the second time. I don't know if that is why I was in hospital longer, or whether there are different methods here. I don't know if this is common in other countries.

The lazy nurse and the angel

Night shifts, of course, are the ones where you most need to be prepared. After my first bladder operation, the very first evening just before the changeover of shifts, I had 'the lazy nurse'. The one for whom everything is too much trouble. The one with the grumpy face and the weight of the world on her shoulders. Obviously I don't know her story, but I do know the other nurses on her shift were carrying her.

Suddenly I started to have serious pain in my bladder. I'm a person who can take a certain amount of pain with stoicism, after all I've had three children. But if I think it's pain with damage, or I don't know what it is, I'm a bit quicker to react. This was off the scale of pain. So I told myself to relax. Weirdly though, the more I relaxed the more painful it became. We called urgently for the nurse, but she said "in a moment." The moments became long minutes and the minutes ticked by and the pain increased. This became the worst pain I have ever experienced and some choice expletives were uttered, believe me. Looking back I could have auditioned for the exorcist! I couldn't speak. I was just flapping my hands at my husband and banging the bed and screaming. Finally, one of the changeover nurses arrived. She was called Johana. She became my angel of mercy. Immediately she realised that my bladder which was being irrigated at the time was literally full to the point of bursting. More saline was entering, but nothing was leaving due to a blockage. Worse still, the more I relaxed the more I was permitting water to flow in. She gently backflushed the tube, and peace was restored. A couple more times during the night the tube became blocked again and Johana had to clear it. The angel of mercy knew straight away what had happened, took a big syringe and made life bearable again. Truth be told, she probably saved my bladder if not my life! This wasn't the last similar problem I would have.

We've always said that water was my nemesis. And so it seems to be. (Stories of my battles with water in both Hull and Andalucia appear in my book Making It Small).

Full 70s?

One of the things which preoccupied me in the early days before diagnosis, was the question of pubic hair. As a girl whose sexual maturity came on in the days of the full 'curly', when the only naked pubis appeared in porno mags, if you weren't sporting pubic hair your doctor might suspect you of having loose morals. I wondered, now, as a woman of nearly 60 whether the medics would consider my now half way 'set' still gross, or whether total removal would still carry a stigma in my age group. Decisions decisions. So I tidied up and shortened some more for all my investigative appointments. I was soon to have the decision taken out of my hands. For my first TURBT along came a nurse with a dry razor and removed most of it, somewhat untidily and certainly uncomfortably for me. Of course from the next TURBT onwards I was prepared and as smooth as a newborn!

Results

I was waiting around 6 weeks between my first TURBT and the results, because of the CAT scan. This was partly my fault because I insisted on a full body scan rather than just the abdomen.

All these unintentional delays, one on top of the other, could have cost me my life. By the time I was diagnosed the cancer had spread through the bladder wall and affected a handful of lymph nodes. I had got to the stage where the decision was, was it worth the extensive operation? What was the likelihood of success? To be honest, I was even worried that, post Brexit, and given the awful attitude of the UK towards Europeans getting free healthcare, that might colour the final decision. People might poohpooh this idea, but if the decision is on a knife edge any health service decides, on the balance between chance of success, and treating a lot more people who stood a greater chance earlier in their illness history. Any small personal bias could sway a decision at such a late stage. My urologist shook his head when he told me the results of the first TURBT and told me it was pretty bad, and the tumour appeared to have invaded the muscle wall of the bladder. We were definitely at the 11th hour. My chances of getting a successful outcome were on that knife edge.

There was discussion even before my second TURBT as to whether they might or might not take my bladder out. My husband, understanding the language, but not grasping the implications, nudged me when he heard this and suggested that the fact they might not have to take it out was hopeful. I shook my head at him sadly. Fortunately, in the end their decision was at least for giving me the second TURBT to clarify my chances. It was like getting to the finals! I know it was still touch and go.

Gone were all my fears of losing my bladder. I was fighting for my chance at life.

Whenever I hear anyone say that they are horrified about the idea of losing their bladder. I ask them to imagine that they too are at the 11th hour, and the choice is to keep their bladder ... or their life. It makes the decision to love the bag so much easier! I love my bag for life and there are some extra benefits too.

For my American readers. We have a healthcare system which is free at the point of need. It is a bit overstretched and you don't get to stamp your foot so much when you aren't paying. That doesn't mean that if you're rich you can't pay for extras or speed, it just means that you don't have to. Not that I could pay anyway, which is a very good reason for having a national health service!

Fight Bladder Cancer group (28 Nov 2016)

From now on referred to as FBC Group

> Hi. Just want to introduce myself and ask for a little support with language if anyone here can help. I'm a Brit living in Spain and have just had a fairly large tumour removed from my bladder along with some smaller ones. I haven't yet had my CAT scan or the Biopsy results. I speak Spanish but not medical Spanish and so far I haven't really got to grips with the jargon even in English especially the abbreviations. As most abbreviations in Spanish are somewhat reversed I wonder if there's a member here who has been through the process of seeing the Oncologist and being offered the various treatments in Spain.

CT Scan - (5th Dec 2016)

I had a CT scan today. I thought they were going to do an MRI but TAC turned out to mean CT. Just goes to show why I needed translation! I'll get all my results in one appointment a week today. I don't expect them to be very low grade because of the size of my primary tumour and the fact there were loads of little ones covering the whole of one side of my bladder.

Meanwhile I'm doing all I can to get myself as healthy as possible ready in case I need further treatment (likely). I'm cutting out sugar because I have a terrible sugar habit. I'm also taking golden drops (turmeric, pepper and coconut oil- homemade) and drinking tea made from ginger, cinnamon, black pepper and cloves. I might be overdoing the black pepper because today my stomach is sore. It could just as easily be the horrible stuff they made me drink for the CT scan. Anyway I'm interested in foods as medicine and always have been. If you're interested in my reasons lookup "Antiangiogenesis" and "Candida and cancer" because I'm not going to preach alternative meds at anyone. This is just part of MY journey. So far the bladder irritation seems to be going in a positive direction though.

CT scan side effects (FBC group 6 Dec)

I had a really bad night last night just itching and twitching and generally feeling irritable after the CT scan. Have had a headache all day today too and I feel as if I've got slightly swollen glands in the back of my neck/base of my skull. I don't know if I've even got any glands there! Anyone else had this reaction to the contrast. That's what I'm assuming has caused it.

Results (FBC Group Nov 2016)

Just had my results. Not great but pretty much what I expected. I think the biopsy and CT results differ on the T level but I've got Grade 3. Offering me removal of bladder and womb. Possibly with a neobladder IF further biopsy shows the urethra will take it. Interested to hear from people who have the neobladder whether they think it was worth it as compared to a stoma. (Has) anyone had both and preferred the stoma? Is it normal for your first results appointment not to contain any discussion of Chemo pre or post op? I did really well with understanding Spanish. I had done my homework. I heard on one of the discussions here that the neobladder op is very long and complex. Is the removal & stoma one as long and as complex?

After this group post I did some research and decided I didn't want a neobladder. The reason for this is that I was worried about going through the whole training myself to use it only to get stress incontinence which would have a real negative effect on my life. I also believe you have to self catheterise and I really didn't fancy that. In the end it turned out that I didn't have the option because my urethra was possibly affected by the cancer too. I was happy that I'd already made that decision. I was also told that even the stoma operation could take up to ten hours and is one of the longest, most complicated and most expensive operations there is. I was going to be very lucky to get one!

Acceptance - Dec 2016

Dear Rosie (Childhood friend) Finally got round to reading and translating my discharge notes yesterday and they defo (definitely) use the word tumour. So that's definitive. The way they describe the size and quality of the main tumour it sounds fairly invasive. They said it was a neoplasm with a firm base or words to that effect. I'm not significantly more nor less frightened by that. I think I've got a sort of mental fog with a central theme of "I told you so." It's a win for me either way really because I love to be proved right (so competitive!) and I'm now at a stage where something can be done ... or if not, at least I know. The only thing better would have been to be proved wrong! Even though we've only recently got to know the adult versions of ourselves, I think you already know I'm coping fine at the moment from my tone. do reserve the right to go through all the other stages. Anger, grief denial, etc. that people threaten you with if any of that becomes useful to me. Especially if the spoiled child within the self-sufficient adult doesn't get her own way. I did have a go at Frank about a thoughtless moment or three on his part just after the op. I had to tell him that when I told him I needed him to be there at a certain time the next day he shouldn't read between the lines that it was OK to be an hour and a half late! Leaving me with only half an hour of support before he had to leave for Madrid. Here everyone has their family in support overnight and at all times ... except me. I'm English, so I don't expect that, but just as there's such a thing as relative poverty there's also relative loneliness. I was lonely. He got both barrels when he got back yesterday!

Go home and enjoy Xmas!

The urologist told me I'd have my second TURBT in January. That seems an awful long time to be sitting with cancer growing inside me of course. I asked him if there was anything I could do to aid my own situation and he said "Just go home and enjoy Xmas," I must admit that even though he meant well, it sounded ominous: like the sort of thing you say when you are pronouncing a terminal prognosis. Fortunately, as I was leaving and as an afterthought, he said "Oh and you could lose a bit of weight ready for the operation." That certainly bucked me up. "I'll do that, even though it's Xmas" I said, and gave him a cheeky grin. At last there was something I felt I could be in control of. I was overweight. Some may say very overweight at ... To be honest I hadn't weighed myself for a while and now I can't remember, so I could have been over 90 Kilos.

I knew the only sure-fire way of me losing weight was to go on a very strict low-carb diet. I'd done it before, years before and very successfully but after a few years of maintaining it, started to pile it on again. I put myself on a high protein plus fat plus fruit and veg diet, with zero grains or potatoes or sugar. I also lowered my milk intake. I had eggs for breakfast and vegetarian garden veg only dishes for tea: often courgette soup. I took to making homemade, almost sugar free custard made with egg yolks and coconut milk and I virtually lived off that with home grown raspberries. I had no chocolate for Xmas, but I did make myself a sugar free Xmas cake which was immensely satisfying served with that same custard. I got so used to low to no sugar I found

I really didn't like sugar on the few occasions when we went out and had to eat what was on offer.

I lost a couple of kilos a week for the first few weeks and then settled to one a week. By the time of my next operation I was already down about 8 kilos! By the RC operation I was under 80 kilos. I was feeling really fit and the eggs seemed to be building my blood back up when I needed it. I then lost another 5 over the next few years and just recently I dropped another four. Now at 66 Kilos which I think is healthy.

I also realised it couldn't harm me to do some gentle exercise. I always had good core strength for a 'chubby' girl, and I knew this was going to be important to me. I forced myself to go out for walks and to do a few gentle tummy exercises. I was getting 'match-fit' and that my outcome was likely to be better for it.

Another thing which I've always done before any surgery is bathed in a bath with Tea tree oil in it. This is because most infections are taken in by the patients on their own skin and anything I could do to minimise that, I was going to do. Another of those things that can't do any harm and might just help.

Fears (FBC group 23 Dec 2016)

> (I) Could use some reassurance today as all the way through this I haven't felt more than the occasional twinge of discomfort except after my first TURBT of course. I'm still 18 days from my second TURBT and I'm really feeling that this thing is growing into the muscle. It's causing me almost constant discomfort now for the last couple of days and of course it's making me nervous. Especially as the Urologist is telling me that a positive result after the next 'op would be if they *DID* decide to go ahead with the removal. That would be if it hadn't spread. Meanwhile until the Spanish Xmas period is all over there's nothing to stop the cancer getting worse on a daily basis. All the delays really do get me down even though I do have quite a positive attitude overall.

Of course I was worried. Looking back I'm surprised I didn't panic more. This is the sort of message that quite a lot of members of this type of group send at some point in their journey. I think this is exactly what support groups like this are for, to be able to offload your fears when you find you can't cope without a little extra empathy.

Writing my Memoir

One of the things which helped me to go through all the stages of grief associated with an aggressive cancer diagnosis was writing my memoir. I already had bits of it written. In fact, I first compiled my father's writings into his memoir. The day after I finished that and published it (new years eve ready for the year of culture in my home city) I had a steep drop in mood and realised that that project had given me something to take my mind off the wait for results and decisions. I needed a new project. I started on my own memoir which I finally published under the title "Making It Small." This was a pun on the twin facts that I'm a miniaturist and also never got rich. The act of writing your life memories down whether or not your condition is terminal is very cathartic and I recommend it to everyone even if it's just to hand on to your children. I certainly had a deeper understanding of my (deceased) Dad after I'd done his.

Workplace exposure (FBC group 29 Dec 2016)

> I'm interested in the subject of what workplace exposures tend to be contributory factors in bladder cancer, but this subject doesn't seem to be talked about here. Is it a taboo? Also it annoys me that doctors always put it down to smoking first. I think this has a tendency to make the sufferer think that it's somehow his own fault and, worse, means little research is done into possible other causes/triggers. I did smoke for about 14 years of my life but have been smoke free for double that time. My history with dye pigments however is very prominent. One of the reasons it took them so long to

diagnose me, I think, is that they didn't take this into account. My previous smoking was immediately noted but not the history with pigments. Since more and more young women it seems are being diagnosed with bladder cancer there must be something else going on. Isn't it down to us current sufferers to discuss these issues and move for more research to be done to save new generations which may include our own children and grandchildren? I know this is a support group primarily, so where do we discuss these things?

What causes cancer?

Some people get angry when you suggest that the appearance of cancer might have something to do with your state of mind because they think you're suggesting that their cancer or that of a loved one might be their own 'fault'. Of course it isn't. To me, it was obvious. Even though I didn't expect to get cancer myself. In fact it was the furthest thing from my conscious mind when it appeared. I thought I'd probably get a heart attack: maybe die of one. That seemed the likely first major illness for someone from my family with my personality type. I'd seen friends of mine of a certain age, who'd seen a sudden or more progressive loss in their lives suddenly find that they had life threatening cancers around 2 years after their crisis. Many died. One friend's son died suddenly. She was distraught. Inconsolable. She followed him out very quickly after discovering her cancer (I didn't hear which type) almost exactly 2 years later. Another friend who'd had a very traumatic childhood, whose mother had been a tyrant and unloving had a serious argument with her own son about his behaviour and drug taking. At this point she decided she had to let go of him, but suffered intensely from guilt and, importantly, hopelessness. Within two years she had brain cancer and two years after that, she died.

There have been other friends whose full story I don't know but in each case they were smokers and or drinkers and in some cases they had a period where they felt hopelessness and/or perhaps abandoned the care of their own mind and body.

I always felt this to be the case, so I asked myself how was it I didn't see my cancer coming and avert it? I don't think we notice when we are treating ourselves badly. We are just trying to do the best we can in difficult circumstances.

I've also seen younger people suffer from terrible losses but in each case either they did not give way to hopelessness, or their youth and good health were still intact enough to protect them. Some older people also lose loved ones but have a positive and healthy mental attitude and or a healthy body to start off with. They grieve and they eventually let go of the pain. They either have the support of their families, very good health or they have no, or less residual guilt or hopelessness.

It seems to me that the latter is the most important. Guilt and hopelessness seem to be very detrimental as they cause you to mistreat yourself. Those, added to a certain age and infirmity either caused by long term poor diet or lack of exercise seem to have cumulative effects which can manifest in the bodies inability to shrug off the cancerous cells which normally live and die naturally inside all of us.

So when I did get cancer, I sort of said to myself "oh yeah ... well why wouldn't I, after those sh**ty years?" Instead of getting confused and angry, I had something else to do.

I believe even people who are very balanced need to look at their mental health when going through cancer or caring for someone, or losing someone from cancer. I needed to get my body fixed but I knew my mind needed a tweak or two too.

Night fears (FBC group 1 Jan 2017)

> How does everyone cope with waking up with bladder discomfort and the brain just clicking into and staying on the "you've got cancer" cycle? Just saying "don't think about it" doesn't work. If anything you're just going to think more about the things you try to get out of your mind. Anyone got any effective hints or tricks? I've lost so much sleep recently!

Second TURBT (FBC group 10 Jan 2017)

I've just been told I'm going in tonight for my second TURBT as I'm first on the list in the morning. On the one hand, it's good to be first on the list. Less chance of cancellation and more chance the surgeons will be sharp (pun not intended). On the other hand I'm not ready! House is a mess, 3 classes to teach in the next few hours. AAArghhhh! (I'm) Now wondering how much work I can get away with taking in for tonight and whether I should re-learn how to play MahJong while I'm in.

In the end I took a notebook and wrote up some of these stories. I knew from the last time I was likely to be in for 5 days. I was such a workaholic I was never happy just lying around if there was anything else I could do. I needed to pack quickly and put my phone, my kindle, my neck pillow and a laptop my brother had given me in the case, so I could write. I also sneaked my travel kettle in and my decaf tea bags!

My roommate this hospital stay was a lady who had come in for her 5th TURBT. She was living with recurrent bladder cancer. Every couple of years they would bring her in and take any new growths out. She seems to be very relaxed about this process having been through it a few times.

Calls of nature

The one thing I would never do if there was any other solution at all, would be to use a bedpan for anything other than a wee. So it was that I ended up two days into my second TURBT stay, having hung on for most of that, forcing a sweet little mature nurse to uncouple me from the irrigation bags and saline drips to let me attend to what, by then, was a fearsome call of nature. I begged and then tried all the other tactics with menaces of doing it myself anyway and not a few tears. Of course the kind-hearted but very competent nurse was not moved at all by my threats, though I am twice her size, but my tears melted her very soft heart. So, risking, as she thought, a dangerous fall which I promised wouldn't happen and certainly wouldn't be on her watch, she allowed me to leave the bed. Basic needs were attended to in very short order and I'm not sure who was the most relieved, me, or her. And I was, believe me, extremely relieved.

Male nurses (in Spain)

How much pain can one slightly sadistic or at least a little impatient nurse inflict, with just a few millilitres of saline? Well, believe me, a lot! All it takes is a recently operated bladder already full to the brim and the push of just one syringe full with slightly more than the necessary force to have you screaming in pain. So that the easy extraction of a tiny blockage in an outflow tube becomes a major and rather frightening procedure.

My catheter kept getting blocked. By now I knew why. There was so much debris in my bladder they just couldn't clear it all out. There were blood clots too. I took to watching these blockages move down the tube into the bag. Sometimes I went to the loo instead of calling the nurse and gave a little 'push' with the little bit of muscular contraction I still had in my poor old bladder. I knew not to push too hard because I could have damaged the wound but it seemed preferable to a careless flush by a nurse. Sometimes the urine bypassed the catheter. Sometimes it shifted the blockage. I was acutely aware of these blockages, and I wasn't going to let one settle in for long!

When the next time the blockage occurs and the nurse refuses to help the pressure can be such that the urine is intent on leaving through force of quantity, a very strong contraction will bypass the blocked tube completely. When the same busy/lazy nurse suggests you just allow it to flow and wet the bed, most of us would rather risk injury to get to the toilet first. The contractions and the subsequent bed wetting becomes preferable to ever allowing an irritated nurse near you with a syringe again. If you are unlucky enough to 'win' the grumpy nurse lottery; and get him again the next time you have a problem in an intimate and very tender area, you realise just how powerless you are.

It's not much help when nurses say, it doesn't matter, they've seen and heard it all, wetting the bed is nothing. Your dignity is precious, and you only want to lose it bit by bit when all else fails. On the other hand when you get an angel of mercy, you value them above gold. So you start to count the shift pattern and, if at all possible, you get any problems solved before the end of a good shift or when you get a bad one you hold on as long as possible until the better nurse comes along.

After this second TURBT I had blockages again. Unfortunately after an entire day of behaving well enough the line got blocked on the night shift. As if to prove my theory that machismo is alive and well and living in Andalusia I drew the short straw once again and got another lazy nurse who this time also happened to be male. He was a bit too rough with the syringe and had me crying out and trying to tell him what the problem was. The next day I told my urologist about this problem and she told me why I must make sure sure it didn't happen again. This time, she said, it was likely to be even more serious than my first TURBT, given that this time they had punched right through my bladder to remove the mass in the muscle and some of the lymph nodes. I was extremely sensitive this time to blockages and any discomfort.

On the night shift once again I was blocked up. Frank had his eye on the bag and wasn't going to let me go an hour without evidence of passing water. Now I'm sure the nurse (yet another male nurse) is a perfectly nice man and very good at his job but he did walk around with an air of superiority: quite literally with his nose in the air. Oh well, I thought, If I explain very carefully what the doctor has told me about the bladder wall being so delicate and likely to rupture if too much pressure is put on it he might understand the reasons I'm 'twittery' after an hour of no urine. Given that I'm drinking so much and my kidneys are clearly working splendidly …

No, I wasn't allowed the time to speak, and received a lecture on how if there is no urine in the bladder no urine will flow. Yes, I said, I know that but there is urine. So how do you know that? He asked me. Well, I have bladder contractions. So he started to explain to me what a sensitive organ the bladder is and how it can contract when there's a foreign body, all very interesting but that didn't explain the piss flowing down my leg because the pressure was so great it was bypassing the tube. Then he started telling me that if you abuse washing the tubes it's a good way to get an infection. All very well and a very good point but if the hole they punched in my bladder gets pressure on it, as my lady urologist explained, there would be much more severe consequences. That's why I was catheterized in the first place. I must admit I have no recollection as to what he said as he walked away but I think it was something about leaving it until there was some urine to flow. I'd already left it well over an hour and I had been told not to take any chances. Well, I snapped at this point.

"If you don't want to do it, I'd rather you didn't. I'll just go to the toilet (which I wasn't allowed to do) and allow the wee to bypass the system as it's going to do in the bed otherwise". I must admit I let a "You guys are so rough" pass my lips. I know he heard that from the other side of the door because he returned with the lovely auxiliary Lola. He said, "OK I'll do it. I'm just saying that you patients think when they take away the irrigation system that urine will still flow continuously." "I'm not even continuing this discussion." I said. "You are treating me like an idiot and I don't want you to touch me anyway because you're angry and I'm angry. I won't be relaxed, and I've already had experience of the ministrations of an overworked male nurse."

By this time I was in tears of frustration, but I think I had 'won the fight' because he let me explain the whole of my history with the dreaded catheter blockages. After all that he did unblock mine. I insisted that Lola stayed with me though. He also found that the tube and bag weren't flowing properly either, because they hadn't been changed in 2 days. He also passed the tube through the correct part of the hanger system. What a blessed relief …

again. So I thought I'd try to make it up to him by showing him that I valued his knowledge, asking him about stoma care. "Why do you want to know?" "Because it looks like I'll be having one." I said. "Oh well worry about that when the time comes you don't need to burden yourself with all that now." Oh gawd! Has he just said "don't worry your pretty little head about that" without even the sweetener of the "pretty"?

"I'm the sort of person who likes to be informed ahead of time. It kind of puts me back in control of my life," I explained. "I might just get an RC and a new chance of life, I'd kind of like to know what I'm in for if I get lucky." "Why do you say that?" He asked. "Because it was an impressively big and aggressive tumor and I thought I'd had my chips." Sorry, I fib here. I said nothing about chips but the dialogue was getting a bit boring. "I could ask my friends in the UK, but the system might be different here." I told him. So he agreed to show me a stoma bag and wafer and I was able to ask about swimming and about whether they were available on prescription. All very important stuff to fill my pretty little head with. So, pretty little head adequately filled with advance information, I had a rapidly filling bag and a less fractious relationship with my nurse for the day at least.

Readers of this may think I have a problem with men. Oh yes, I do, but not the one you might think. I like them, too much for my own good maybe. I love intelligent conversations with men and if anything I prefer male company to female. I'm a bit of a bloke I suppose. I'm perfectly happy to be treated like a lady. However, that doesn't and never has included in any sense that the word lady, especially when combined with 'old' might be equated with 'idiot'.

I blame the parents. It's a long cultural history to unpick. Even my friend Montse behaves like it's a man's world, cleaning her able-bodied divorced Dad's house for him because he won't do it for himself.

Anyway, the change in this guy's bedside manner towards me was obvious from then on. He realised that I wasn't a 'silly old woman,' and I hope that he'll forever drop the mansplaining manner towards his more mature patients ... but I doubt it. It still seems to be ingrained in Spanish culture. Anyway, this nurse and I subsequently became friends and whenever he was on a shift he came for a chat and brought me oranges from his garden and we chatted about garden herbs and aromatherapy. It turns out he was a particular fan of lavender.

Decision time

I knew that, because of the late stage of my cancer, the decision whether to operate hung on a knife edge and I was determined to let the urologist know that I had a great quality of life and that I was going to be worth saving if it were at all possible. By this time the 'cancer bonus' had kicked in. By that I mean the absolute knowledge that life is short and valuable and worth fighting for and that I personally had a value. I was glad I was 59 and hadn't quite reached that other psychological tipping point.

I'd apologised to my own body for being a lazy and careless little sh** and I knew that I could give 100% to my second life if I got the chance. It was a nervous wait.

I hung on the urologist's every word for signs of hope. On the 4th day he told me that the decision had been made. They were booking me in for a full day in surgery. I was going to have removal not only of the bladder but also of the womb, cervix, appendix and some lymph nodes. I'm sure some people would find that a horrifying prospect ... I was ecstatic! If I'd thought drinking was a good idea at the time I'd have popped a bottle of cava.

There is nothing like being 'borderline' for surgery to fix your attitude to the whole idea.

I now tell anyone who is unsure whether they want an RC when it's been offered, to ask themselves how they would feel if the offer was suddenly withdrawn.

My urologist told me that they would give me a 'Bricker' ileostomy, which meant they were going to take a part of my intestine and repurpose it as a passage to take urine from the ureters (from the kidneys) out through a stoma, a little hole on my belly just to the right of and a little below my navel. The only reason they weren't doing it immediately was that my body had already been through so much and I needed to regain my strength and build some new blood. I was booked in for a fortnight later. I had work to do!

Lymph nodes (FBC group)

I had my second TURBT a week ago on Tuesday, they took out a deeply embedded 5cm tumour but couldn't get all the roots as they were very deep. I believe they also punched through to biopsy the lymph nodes. I lost quite a bit of blood, and they kept me in a week. They have decided to take out my bladder which is very good news for me. Sent me home for just 2 weeks to recover my blood levels and then back in and then "the biggie." In the end I'm glad I got used to the idea of having a stoma because, as I thought, the urethra does look likely to be affected at some point if it was left in.

Apparently German for bladder cancer is blasenkrebs. I don't know if that sounds even worse? In Spanish, bladder is vejiga pronounced vehiga … There now, you've learned two new languages today.

Feeling 'Waspish' (FBC Group 9 jan 2017)

How do other women who are at, or nearing what was the old retirement age coping with not being able to retire and having to claim benefits instead when they are unwell? Under the old system I'd have been able to retire in April. Now, If I were in the UK I'd have got sickness benefit. As an expat I don't even get that fallback. Since my husband's work pretty much relies on mine this put us in a very difficult place. The changes were supposed to be to give 'equality' but we 50s women had never had equality of opportunity, certainly not the kind of equality that lets you build up a pension in the short time after the childcare years. I'm falling through a very big crack right now. It's not even being taken from us to give the money back to the people. It's to feed it upwards. Excuse my rather political Grrr moment please.

People in the UK seemed to assume that there were benefits coming in, but there was nothing, except the help of those who were particularly thoughtful or aware. Eventually I had to ask some people. It was both humiliating and educating. I became sensitive to 'strings attached' and 'no strings attached' help. I was very surprised and moved by the latter and sometimes had to shrug off feeling humiliated by the former. One thing I wasn't going to do was take lectures on the fecklessness of artists! This was the new me and I wasn't taking, or giving myself any of that sh**.

Pre-ops for Radical Cystectomy (30 Jan)

I spent most of today racing around trying to find someone to give me a flu jab, which I was told I should have before the operation. No luck at all. The local nurse wasn't at all interested in my problem and he wouldn't call the hospital (where I'd just been sent to him from) to discuss where else I should try. In the end I went back the 10 km into the hospital and managed to catch my consultant urologist again before he finished his shift. It was he who picked up the phone and called the ward. They said they would have one ready for me when I go in tomorrow. A bit last minute, but I certainly can see the sense in being vaccinated against getting a flu when I'm at my weakest.

Apparently tomorrow I am going to have my intestine filled with odour-free nutrition-free gel. I have been told in advance, not to eat anything interesting tomorrow. It's no fun being told all your favourite healthy food is off the menu. Especially when you know for the next week you won't see a vegetable, nor a piece of fruit!

The members of this forum who've had an RC, followed by what's known as a 'Bricker' will already know what I'm talking about. They're cleaning out my intestines ready to take a piece out to form my stoma. Do they do that for all stomas? All I can think of is how the women in the village clean out the pig intestines after a 'matanza' to make the sausages. I may never look at a 'morcilla tonta' or a sausage the same way again!

Pre op nerves (FBC group 31 Jan)

> I'm just wobbling a bit today. I'm going in for all the pre-treatments before tomorrow's big RC with removal of all the other useless bits. Apparently they're leaving my brain in though! My immediate family are all back in England. Well, one's snowboarding in France. Although I've told them I don't need them here I do feel relatively alone compared with all the other people in the hospital who have their relatives around all the time. (This is normal in Spain) I've told my husband to get a good night's rest too for the long day tomorrow. But when people ask me where my family are, I can't help welling up, and feeling very lonely. Has anyone got any coping mechanisms for this please?

Many people on the bladder cancer forum talk about being afraid of the operation. I just wasn't. I think I had got my head around the idea that this was something I was lucky to have the chance of given the advanced nature of my disease. I knew that I was either going to wake up, or I wasn't. Most likely I was, but I was still surprised when I did. I was told later that I'd had a team of 3 actual surgeons working on me in shifts rather than robotic surgery. Well they were double quick. I was told I was in surgery just 6 hours.

The first days after the operation

I woke up groggy and just processed the movements rolling on and off trolleys. I'd forgotten what I was told about being taken to the Intensive Care Unit, but I realised I was on my way somewhere. Frank was there. "I'm alive!" I said, barely processing the idea that there must have been some fear of dying on the operating table. Oh, there's Angeles. "I'm alive, Angeles!" And Montse.

"I'm alive!" It was all I could say. I felt elated but weak: terribly weak. I was aware of Frank being shooed out of the ICU room. It was all beeps and buzzers and I had a tube up my nose into my throat. It made me gag and swallow and swallow and swallow, albeit feebly. The noise. The light! The staff made no attempt to keep the noise down, and the noise was painful. No-one was by my side for most of the time. No one to ask if they could please be quiet. Occasionally someone, unsmiling, would come in and check my monitors, my levels of something or other, or take my blood. Then joy! Frank came back. I had no idea what day it was but I suppose it was the same day. Someone asked Frank to leave the room and they took my tube out. Then someone else passed me a child's toy. I always like presents but I was a little confused. Three blue balls in little chambers. I was told to suck, or was it blow it? My Spanish was hazy. I was shown a mouthpiece and then the person was gone. I blew weakly ... nothing. I felt dizzy. I sucked and the balls wobbled. Frank returned and I did my cheerful 3 year old act for him and showed him my new toy, blowing and sucking till something moved and then, exhausted by the effort I gave up. Angeles returned, but it was too painful to speak to anyone. I don't mean physically painful. I mean mentally and emotionally exhausting. All I wanted was Frank's hand and his stroke of my head which is the best medicine in the world! Too soon he was gone again: thrown out by my jailers.

This was the start of 48 hours in purgatory. Of course I was dimly aware of a rising ache in my lower abdomen, but the pain killers were supplied if I asked for them and I felt the blessed relief wash over me so I could sleep a little. The next day I was more conscious, even though the night was endless and seemed sleepless. I was bed bathed, with scratchy soapy blue and white pads which I came to love, ready for the consultant's visit. Then they smiled at me, it seemed for the first time, and lathered me with some oil to keep my skin from sores. I wanted to tell them how horribly oxygenated the oil smelled, but I just thanked them for their care. By this time I was aware of my stoma and the two tiny tubes which were presumably diverting the urine past my newly constructed (Bricker) ileostomy. These passed directly into the plastic pouch attached by a ring of brown, hardened gum to my right abdomen and on into a night bag on the side of the bed. I took tentative peeks at the little bulge of pink sprouting from my belly. It was smaller than I had imagined and less frightening. It looked to have been well made even at that point. Instead of calling it 'Gucci', which was my first idea, I named it 'Raspberry'. I had taken time before my surgery to get used to the idea and had even said goodbye and thank you to my bladder for its years of good service before it finally succumbed to having been dreadfully abused by a sedentary lifestyle, chemical toxins and not enough water. I'd decided in advance to welcome my stoma as a lifesaver and not allow myself to feel that it was second best or some kind of punishment.

On the second day I was holding back from screaming. I had to get out of the endless insistent beeping and the staff talking at full volume. My favourite urology consultant returned: everyone hushed. Seeing that one of my tubes was slipping out, took a needle and thread and simply sewed it onto the skin at the side of my stoma with no anaesthetic. And I let him! Maybe I was too weak to care. Maybe I appreciated the silence. The nurses were not the only ones in awe of this quiet mild mannered man. The nurses knew I was weak and kept anxiously checking my blood levels. At some point I was given a bag of plasma. Frank told me on his next visit that I'd lost several pints of blood during the operation and that I'd already received 2 pints during or after the operation. That certainly didn't seem like enough.

After the second night, I was told that I going to be moved to the ward. I could hardly bear the wait. The day crept by mercilessly until oh joy! The porter came for me. Double joy, I was wheeled into a single room. That meant I had no neighbours. Even better, no neighbour's family members. Peace at last! Peace and a better dose of my husband's company.

I will always be grateful for the ICU or UCI as it's called in Spain. But it was hell.

On the ward

Frank visited twice a day rather than having someone with me all the time as Spaniards here normally do. Frank had to take my English classes, or we wouldn't eat! It was a really tough time for him because he had to do all the business work, all the classes and the visits. Angeles and Montse visited every few days which helped a lot and I was really happy to see another friend Inma too. In fact it was Inma's style of quiet, amiable company I craved.

I don't know if they put me in the isolation ward because they took pity on me, or on the other inmates. Not only was it a trial for me sharing, with the constant machine-gun Spanish, for them it must have been annoying having to share with a miserable looking social-phobic Englishwoman. I was far too tired to put on my amiable exterior.

My daughter visited me at this stage. Frank went to pick her up at the airport and I got a phone call from him. Did I have our credit card? What?! Apparently he'd been pulled over in Portugal with a demand for unpaid tolls. We'd always paid our tolls, but the cards hadn't always worked on the telephone system so hadn't always registered. This phone call was physically and mentally painful. I could hardly move, let alone speak. I was so weak and tired. There was nothing I could do and it was so worrying because my daughter was going to be at the airport on her own if he didn't get out of this predicament.

I don't know how he managed to persuade them to take an amount less than the full fine which we didn't have access to, but somehow he got to the airport and got my daughter back to me.

While he was away, I was given another pint of blood, and one more of plasma. Well, it must have been Andalucian blood because within an hour I was full of alegria and ready to fiesta! Not only that, I've always thought that whoever it came from must have had an appetite for walking followed by a cold beer. Neither of which I'd ever had any interest in before then!

My daughter's visit meant the world to me. We'd had some rocky years during her teens and early 20s, but there was something about the switch in the power balance which unpicked years of misunderstandings at a stroke. She could only stay 2 days and so opted to spend the nights with me and the day in between getting washed and fed and some extra sleep. This was just perfect, and I just loved her company. It was like a big girl sleepover! Too soon the visit was over, and a very good friend took her back to the airport for me since there was no chance of my husband driving back into Portugal again with a noose hanging over his head!

Healing

Of course it took a while before my belly stopped looking like a badly punctured, half deflated, beach ball full of dirty looking, bruised holes. I took another peek at my stoma, and I felt then, and am even more sure now, that I got seriously lucky with my surgery team. I had the first urologist as a surgeon who, I believe, actually did the gynaecological bits, and two young women, one of whom was the daughter of the older surgeon. The 'girls' did the ostomy work. It was like a family enterprise. When we had met before and again after, the girls came across as very friendly and not stuck-up and distant at all. They were clearly also very professional, though.

My local hospital is a small community hospital and they didn't have access to a big robotic set up, so my surgery was very much old school and human-hands-on.

I have to say in all the pictures of stomas I've seen I have never seen a more carefully constructed one. I'm sure if there were stoma beauty pageants, mine would certainly make the line-up. I feel very grateful for that, because it made it easier to learn to love my stoma. I think you have to do that anyway because, if you practise a bit of gratitude, it makes the whole process of acceptance and recovery easier. I was, and still am genuinely very grateful for my little 'raspberry-button'. Of course for most of us, the idea of having a bright pink piece of gut sticking out of our belly is initially a bit horrific. Honestly, It's so much easier if you give it a name. I even talk to it like a naughty child on the occasions when it misbehaves and pees all over during changes.

It was really weird the first time I looked at it when I was naked in the bath and saw its little 'crawly' contractions. I quickly flipped 'weird' into 'funny' in my mind. It's all a matter of perception. I now bath with my bag on, as we bathe in untreated water from a well.

If you are grossed out by it you will have a harder time. I decided consciously to 'make friends' with it and in my opinion that's the best way to get to the acceptance stage of your new reality.

An important consideration is where the surgeon will place your stoma. We had had a discussion and I pointed to where I wanted it. That's exactly where they put it. I got lucky because I didn't really know much about it. Mine was put approximately 5cm to the right and 5cm down from my navel. I'm grateful for that positioning, because it doesn't get squeezed or rubbed by my waistband. The drawback is that the 'tap' at the bottom of the bag does sit, sometimes uncomfortably, at the top of my leg, but it's easily repositioned without any embarrassment just by a little movement of the bag.

'Blanda Facil' - Feb 2017

For about 5 days I wasn't allowed to eat. I was craving food even though I was being given all the nutrition I needed through a drip. I'm not sure if this long wait is common but it seems that here at least they want to know that your gut has healed and is truly ready for work again. Ah well. Looking for the upside, at least, I thought, this was going to be good for my weight loss program! And in fact it did seem to calm my food cravings.

It probably won't surprise anyone when I say that the food in the Spanish hospital was as dreadful as UK ones. Not that each individual item was so bad, just that, as a combination the subset

"Blanda Facil" (bland and easy - presumably to digest) consisted of white, cream and brown coloured foods and, except on one day, absolutely nothing in the line of vegetables. I was craving veggies from about 2 days in and fats, the hospital system also seems to be hanging on to the outdated idea that all fats are bad for you. Only one day of a 16 day stay did I have a really nice meal. Two place fillets and veg, and a lovely baked apple. Oh and the ubiquitous thin tasteless bone broth and a roll.

The breakfast was always a bread roll and 2 packs of butter, and one of jam. I always refused the bread roll etc and just took the decaf coffee (no tea option in Spain) and some fruit illegally smuggled in by my husband. In fact a large part of my diet was tubs of berries. By the 5th day on 'Blanda Facil' I was craving something fatty or oily. I decided that I'd have a small amount of bread and a large amount of butter for breakfast. Unfortunately I was to be thwarted again as the butter wasn't. It was margarine. I certainly wasn't going to be eating margarine with my new attitude to looking after my diet!

Eventually, a couple of days before they let me out I'd complained about the blanda facil menu so much that some kind nurse had put me down for a special instead. The paper said "abundante verduras" (lots of veg). That evening my veg came. A great mountain of courgettes and a salad. Plus the horrid broth. This time lentils (unsalted of course). The next lunch time a mountain of green beans and a tomato salad with the thin soup with chopped egg and ham in the bottom. Ugh!

Kidney pain

I still had the little tubes directly into my kidneys. The nurses were still changing my bag for me daily. There were little taps on the tubes which they turned off to change the bag. One day I started to get pain in my back after a change. I didn't connect the dots though, until I was in agony. Coincidentally it was my Angel nurse Johana who sorted this out again. The nurse who had changed my bag had forgotten to turn the taps on again after the change and the pain was pressure in my kidneys. The positive in this was that I now knew exactly what kidney pain was, and exactly where you felt it. If I have a kidney infection, chill or blockage in the future I'll know what it is because of the location of the pain.

A rebel without a coffee

Once I'd been in hospital a couple of weeks and I felt really well, apart from the final healing of the lower part of my "belly zipper" which, annoyingly, had to be undone again to drain a haematoma. The wind pains and the grumbling reorganisation of my intestines was making the normal digestive/excretion routine a little slow and painful. I realised that I was missing an early morning coffee and although I'd mostly given up on sweet things, a rather sickly Nescaf' cappuccino from the machine in the basement seemed to be the only thing that could quite hit the spot. The Hospital breakfast didn't arrive until around 10 in the morning and their 'café con leche de sobre' (meaning a packet of coffee sprinkled on to a cup of lukewarm milk) arrived a little too late. "Old Grumpy Guts", and here I'm referring to my actual lower intestine and not to my early morning mood, needed a kick start to get its morning thing out of the way to be comfortable and relaxed. At first I pleaded for assistance or at least a blind eye to my leaving the ward. A couple of times I did get someone to walk down with me. On the third day, not finding a free member of staff, I decided to go feral. Just for safety's sake I told someone's daughter what I was about to do and to tell on me if I wasn't back within 5 minutes. I was back in two and in the toilet ten minutes later! I should also mention that for quite a while after the operation the wind pains can be pretty intense. Whatever doesn't travel out through your guts does seem to have to be reabsorbed. And that takes time.

Abdominal support - Feb 2017

They fitted me with an abdominal support belt pretty quickly after I got out of bed. That thing was a real boon. It meant I could move more and, touch wood, I never have had a hernia although I have had some 'threats'. There have been odd feelings where I've felt something trying to get through my abdomen wall. There's one site near my stoma where I feel this and one under my ribs. Each time, as soon as I feel that crawly movement, I sit up straight and gently let it move back into place before tightening my muscles again.

Home! ... Not home

Getting home was both joyous ... and hard. My feeling of fatigue was so painfully intense and I had so many things to remember. Simply changing my bag was hard but changing the wafer seemed like climbing a mountain. I knew that the road to recovery was not going to be an easy or a quick one.

Unfortunately a few days later I was back in hospital again. I'd been back to have my kidney tubes taken out and when I went home I started to feel very strange. I think I vomited and had diarrhea but to be honest I can't remember exactly. Certainly I was sweating and febrile. We went back to the emergency room and I was admitted for another few days. This time I wasn't lucky enough to have my private room and so I was desperate to get out again. Apparently this reaction to the removal of the tubes is not uncommon.

I also had to go back several times to have my haematoma checked and drained and some interesting ultra absorbent material packed into the wound. It made the bottom part of my scar just a little scruffier than it would have been. Fortunately it's now covered by my now re-grown pubic hair.

Wafer changes, leaks etc.

At first I had to be cautious about changing my wafer (the ring that sticks around the stoma and takes the bag in a 2 part system). Because everything was tender, and I didn't want to risk any damage. I think it's common to all ostomates at first that the belly is misshapen and it's difficult to get a good, leak-free, seal at first. This did give me some tearful sessions at first, and I thought I'd never get it right. I cried to my husband that I didn't want to be 'a pissy old lady'! There was no stoma specialist support and no McMillan nurses for me in Spain, so I just had to get on with it. Fortunately, I'm a problem solver. I found that there were extra sticky strips available so I got a prescription for those. I added more to the leaky side of my undulating belly. I rolled up extra large sanitary towels to use as absorbent pressure pads in the concave area of my belly, inside a pair of large but reasonably tight briefs. This compensated for the awkward dip on one side. For one month I also used a concave wafer until the shape of my belly settled down. Soon I was looking much slimmer and sleeker anyway and as the healing completed I found I could be less cautious when sticking the wafer on. I use the Coloplast Alterna comfort system, and I like it. The wafer has a ridged 'concertina' edge which, as you run a finger round it, firmly 'grabs' the skin. The adhesion seems actually to improve with time. I also use a cotton pad to press the glue inside the clip ring round the edge of the stoma.

Do I smell?

One thing you have to be aware of is that urine through an urostomy smells different. It can often be sulphurous. This is because it's passing through a bit of repurposed gut and the gut still does some of the same jobs. It doesn't know it's now just a urine carrier! It continues to produce mucus. At first a little bit gross until you get used to it. That mucus and the breakdown of the inner edges of the wafter can be a bit sticky to clean up and of course you can worry that you might smell, especially as the wafer stays on for a few days. I believe that my routine prevents this although I only have my husband's word that it works.

Here in Spain I can have up to three changes of bag a day if I really want to. That's because I live in a hot country. I tend to stick to the one change a day though. I don't live in a humid area. I change the wafer after between 5 days and a week. I do my bag change after my bath, which I have each and every night with my bag on. I have never had a problem with this at all. Although I fill the bath to just under the line of my belly, I'm not careful to keep it dry. I imagine in humid areas you probably have to be more aware of how wet you get.

When I change the bag, I use rose water on a cotton wool cosmetic pad. It's a nice, sweet smelling, very mild astringent which is ideal for the job and feels like a luxury but works out very cheap in fact. I also use it for washing my skin between wafer changes. So far, touch wood, in 4 and a half years I have never had an infection. Sometimes you literally have to pick the old glue off your skin, but I find that's only in the bit immediately below my stoma where the urine dissolves the glue more.

Unbroken nights! (FBC Group Feb 2017)

I'm already finding upsides to the urostomy. I can demand a late night cuppa from my hubby knowing that he can't make the excuse that the extra fluids will keep me up tonight! Oh the joy of an unbroken night's sleep! One of my elderly female relatives is having real problems with urinary incontinence. That's a future I will never have to face now. After three big babies that had, until then, been on the cards for my future. Another reason for gratitude.

I finally got round to telling my friends and customers on Facebook etc what was going on. Mostly I preferred to carry on as normal, but there came a time when it was going to be obvious and a proper announcement was better than letting people gossip. Some people prefer to let everyone know all the way through their journey. I didn't. What I lost in support I gained in freedom from bland 'prayers' messages, which would have driven me mad! The villagers already knew because of village gossip.

Telling the world (on my Facebook page)

Dear Friends. I've been holding out on you all a few months, and I know it might seem that I've been a bit uncommunicative. I've missed some (miniatures) fairs and haven't fully explained myself. Sorry! I've been battling a very aggressive bladder cancer. I had decided to keep it a temporary secret for several reasons. The major one was because I'm very independent, and an atheist I didn't want any sympathy or prayers however well meaning. I just wanted to get on with finding out whether I had any chance of a cure. And if not, enjoy any time left! We also had to put most of our effort into hospital visits, operations, etc. What time was left we had to spend earning enough just to get by. Things were a bit tough, and I was feeling a bit sorry for myself at times. At other times I was feeling super positive. I believe this is a normal enough reaction. My family and those friends I did tell were fantastic and supportive.

Well, it was touch-and-go for a while whether it had just gone too far. I had two removals of cancer from my bladder, but that wouldn't ever be the end of it. The second one showed deep muscle invasion. So no chance of removal leaving my bladder intact. I finally got the news I wanted to hear. If they really got a move on and performed a radical cystectomy (bladder, womb, ovaries, appendix, lymph nodes, etc.) I would have a good chance of beating the cancer.

I've just come out of hospital after all this was done, leaving me almost half the woman I was! (only joking), but practically cancer free! As a precaution I'm likely to have a short course of chemotherapy. I feel like I've been given a second life! Here's my challenge to my friends. If you want to reply, please try finding a greeting that doesn't use either the words 'sorry' or 'prayers. 'OK? There are going to have to be some radical changes in my work life too. I have some quirky ideas going on about how to make my daily bread from now on. So watch this space! Frank will of course continue to run the business.

Night Sweats (FBC group)

Can anyone advise how long the night sweats last after RC with hysterectomy & appendectomy? Any tricks to reduce them? Mine usually start at 4 or 5 in the morning and continue until I get up, so could be related to blood sugar levels and hormone activity???

I got lots of replies about surgical menopause. A bit too late for that! Many people said it lasts quite a long time. I don't remember when that stopped ... But it did.

There was also a little problem of discharge for a few months. That stopped eventually too.

Bicarb' (FBC group 4 March)

Some advice please. I have a 'team' of urologists, and they disagree. One says I should be on bicarbonate of soda to keep the acidity of my blood down, and he prescribed it for me. The other quite fiercely contests this, and she wouldn't give me a prescription when they sent me home. (I have a 'Bricker' urostomy).

Nobody seemed sure of this one, but I do sometimes take bicarb when I feel as if I'm a bit 'toxic. ' By toxic I mean that I have certain symptoms including very itchy feet and hands and underarms etc. from time to time. I put that down to needing a bit of a clean out and I clean up my eating (no sugar or alcohol or chocolate) and I take some bicarb for a few days.

My mother's generation used to take 'liver salts' (magnesium and bicarbonate of soda) when they felt what they used to call "liverish".

The Day Hospital

The first chemotherapy treatment was strange. The Day Hospital had been renovated and had a space age silent white automatic sliding door. It was like stepping into another world. There were a dozen cubicles to provide just a little privacy. I felt like a fraud because by this time I was feeling so well and I still had my hair. It was strange to walk in and sit down and not really feel like one of the patients. Also I was damned if I was going to sit for 5 or 6 hours doing nothing, so I took the first draft of my memoirs in and Frank and I went through them. I seemed to be the only one not staring into the distance. I was told to drink plenty of water and so I did. I was also given an anti-nausea medication before the infusions of which there were three or four, two to defray the side effects of the other two.

The worst part of it was trying to find veins that hadn't been thoroughly damaged by the total of four recent surgeries. I think in the end they had to use the back of my hand, which was annoying for my reading!

I went straight back home and gave the last class to two lovely ladies who'd come over from England. It was OK. I was tired, but nausea hadn't kicked in yet. Over the next couple of days, though I turned into a 'chemo zombie'. I stayed in bed and watched TV or slept. I couldn't bear the taste of anything including plain water which tasted of chemicals. In fact grape and peach juice or pineapple juice were all I could tolerate. When I could eat anything at all it had to be very small and very strongly flavoured. My friend Inma, whose own daughter had been through months of chemo, brought me a homemade fish pate based on anchovies, tuna and mayonnaise. Weirdly I could eat that on rye bread. My weight loss goal was getting closer of course!

Chemo side effects (FBC group 17 Mar)

> Hi. Back for more advice. I don't get much info here in Spain and if I don't understand I'm a bit lost. I'm on my first

week of Gem-cis intravenously. First treatment was Thursday. Apparently I just get one of them the second week in the cycle. Of course I have nausea. Does it improve at all after a few days and is it a bit better with just the one drug? It's bearable: but only just. I'm getting very tired and itchy too.

My 60th Birthday April 2017

I had a wonderful introduction back into life in the form of my 60th birthday 'surprise' party trip. No, it wasn't really a surprise. Only the destination was. If you've got to 60 and nobody has ever thought to throw you a party, surprise or not, it's definitely time to demand one, especially if there's even a small chance it may be your last. I had demanded mine. I stated very firmly that for once in my life I didn't want to be part of the organisation at all. I wanted 'my day' and I needed for others to take the strain for once. It was like a rite of passage into old age.

Apparently there was some discussion between the guests as to whether it was worth making plans before my operation. Hell yes! If not now when? If I hadn't made it through I would still have wanted them to have the party!

My family took me to Lanzarote and, unfortunately, mostly had to pay for it. Frank borrowed some money to pay for our accommodation. He was supposed to have been saving up for a year for it. I'd got enough money together, by not paying bills, for us to have 50 euros a day spending money but it was not all inclusive so that really didn't go far especially when the family wanted to eat out. Money was always too tight. In spite of that, in the end it was just wonderful. It was a revelation to be able to leave the organisation to everyone else. When you've spent your whole life taking responsibility for all your actions and all their outcomes it's the best present in the world and absolutely vital for me to feel that sense of being free from responsibility. I still was not out of the woods. It could still have been my swansong.

We had a lovely time. Members of my family who I didn't expect and hadn't seen for a few years came. I was just out of nausea from my first round of chemo and was feeling great and celebratory. My son said to me "Blimey Mum. You must be the only person who can look better after cancer and during chemo than before." I knew I did.

We had a laugh about the idea of losing my hair as I asked my family to bring me cheap silly wigs. My sister brought me three Disney style wigs which were great fun. Thankfully this was NOT my last birthday either.

Travel with a stoma

People seem to get very nervous about travelling with a stoma. Yes, the new machines can detect your bag and sometimes if you've been standing in line a while after downing a whole 2 litre bottle of water (not wanting to waste it by throwing it out when water is so expensive on the plane!) Honestly, just say "I have a stoma" if you get pulled out of the line to be frisked. If they insist on seeing that it actually is what you say, ask to be taken to a private room or just give them a sneaky peek at the top edge if you're feeling brazen. I do! After all you lost all your dignity in the hospital and airport security have seen it all before and if they haven't it's probably high time they did!

Oh and clothing. You don't need to worry about this either. Mostly your ring and bag are much less visible than you think. I used to wear extra layers to make the line smoother, but now I just make sure I don't wear tight, single colour items. Everything else is just fine, barring swimming costumes but I don't even care about those, these days. There's something very freeing about learning that what other people think of your stoma, is their problem: short of getting it out and waving it about, of course.

3rd Chemo cycle

Really suffering from my 3rd cycle of chemotherapy. Cisplatin/Gemcitabine Anyone else had neuralgia/ neck ache/headache. What did you do about it? Is there permanent damage? The nausea is much worse this time too, I get auditory disturbance and my face feels weird and kind of numb. I also now have a very weird cough that comes in spasms. I don't know if it's related to the chemo. It started while I was away in Lanzarote.

My cousin who had Lyme disease and is very knowledgeable about B12 not only told me I definitely needed B12 and folic acid (together) but explained to me why. Certain medications make you very short of it including Chemo which I was having, Lansoprazole, which I was on and Metformin which I wasn't. She bought me my first batch which was extremely thoughtful. In the future I'd like to try and give something useful to each person I know who is going through cancer treatment, wherever, possible because of the important ways my friends helped me.

I had four rounds in total of chemo, but they dropped the Cisplatin entirely for the 4th round as it seemed to be damaging me too much. On my last day of chemo, I was vomiting, even just on the Gemcitabine. I think it was more a psychological reaction than physical.

Thoughts on Chemotherapy

I'm not going to say that Chemo was not the best thing for me to do at the time. It was. There were several reasons why I opted to do it. Mostly the fear that if I didn't do it I would die. Another important consideration (to me) was: If I don't do it and the cancer comes back in short order, my family would say, "We told her to … but she didn't listen!" I would hate for that to be the thing they most often said about me at family discussions!

It was a strategy with risks though. I knew then, but not as well as I know now, that the side effects of chemo are potentially as bad as the few cells that may have lived to fight another day. Nevertheless, I did have chemo, and I'm out of the other side of it. At first I was weakened but alive. The side effects diminished over the years since, but I still do have some. Vitamin B12 and Folic acid seemed to be a bit of a magic bullet for my side effects of facial neuropathy and tinnitus. A weird allergy-triggered spasmodic cough that arrived just after my first course of Chemo, has never gone away.

In the same position I would have chemotherapy again to kill the cancer completely. However, I can say personally I probably wouldn't have it for short-term life extension, if I had a terminal prognosis. The time feeling sick and other damaging side effects wouldn't be my choice for a very short extra time. That's a current personal belief. Nobody can make those final decisions for you. Maybe I will change my mind if that day comes.

Housework!

I noticed that the only time in my life that my house was clean and reasonably tidy was when I gave up work simply to get over my cancer. Psychologically I was in no mood for anything but the mundane repetitive tasks of cleaning and tidying. I was cleaning and decluttering my mind and my surroundings. Partly of course it was cleaner because there simply was no DIY going on and partly because there were fewer miniatures tools and materials around the place. When I felt creative I simply wrote down my ideas and very often simply passed them to Frank to realise. This has very much become a new post cancer pattern for us. I was worried about how Frank would make a living during and after whatever was to come, if I couldn't. Frank isn't a natural go-getter type but can certainly go and get if he is pointed in the right direction. He is a natural at supporting the creative arts with his abilities with the tech, though. He is a natural realiser of ideas. I'll keep having those until I physically or mentally can't.

Emotionally battered

As I've hinted at before, one of the things we had to cope with, living as we did in Spain, was pretty extreme poverty during my cancer. We had already been in trouble before, but cancer tipped us into an abyss. I don't want to go into the deprivations, nor the pain that we felt when there was nothing, and how difficult it was to ask for and then be refused help. I did realise that I also needed emotional support to cope with the mental turmoil and to allow myself to let go. I needed to allow those who wanted to, to shoulder some of the burdens. And those who didn't, to be respected for or in spite of that decision. I had always been a 'strong woman' but sometimes in the past that had been a mask for having to shoulder burdens that shouldn't have been entirely mine. I never knew how to ask for help and so I wasn't used to rejection either.

I decided to ask my doctor to send me to a therapist. I very much encourage anyone to do this. It wasn't even the actual two sessions with a therapist that helped as much as it was giving myself permission to be in need. It gave me the feeling that I needed space and time to work through how I was in my old life and how I intended to be in my new one. The most important thing I told myself was that I had a value, and the only person that was ever going to put a stamp on that value was me, and that anyone who didn't recognise that value. Well, that was their choice. Maybe even their loss. I wasn't going to give myself any more sh** to deal with.

A sneaky wee (June 2017)

My re-entry into the outside world was for a visit to our favourite Paris (Miniatures) fair. It happened to be the last put on by that organisation and one of our favourites, so I didn't want to miss it. I soon found out another upside of having a bag, especially if you fly 'cattle-class' with Ryanair, which, of course, we did. The bus from the airport took so long to get through the Paris traffic that my bag looked like it could burst at any moment and was incredibly heavy and ugly to carry around. As soon as we got off the bus, I took advantage of the fact that nobody was looking at anybody in that huge throng of people pressing their way towards the metro. I just turned my back to them and emptied my bag into a bush. If anyone saw? Well, I thought, It's just a bit less embarrassing than having a catastrophic failure of the bag or its ring! And certainly I spent that journey in a lot less discomfort than poor Frank.

A brush with 'Natural Medicine'

I was suffering from chemotherapy side effects, and a pharmacist had cautioned me that the two drugs I'd been prescribed for nausea and the neuralgia were more damaging than some honest to goodness cannabis which is legal for medicinal use in Spain. I managed to get a bit from a dispensary in Seville. I think a lot of the medicinal users … aren't. My personal opinion is that taking cannabis acquisition away from illegality is much healthier than making people get closer to the world of illegality just to get a little 'medicine'. I was very wary about how much I used and really knew very little about what was available. I had asked for something that was high in CBD and very low in THC. I used it extremely lightly but it did seem to work. When I went to England, I was going to be without. I didn't mind too much, as I was getting over the side effects of the chemo, but a young friend brought me some 'medicine' there anyway. Of course it is illegal in the UK but I was prepared to have an excuse to show solidarity with my friend. I hadn't used it for 40 years apart from my lightweight medicinal variety that I'd just tried in Spain (I'm over 60). I never did like getting high, because I used to have a tendency to paranoia 'under the influence', but had a little puff or two anyway as I was feeling in safe hands. It was a little weird as we rolled up a tobacco-free mini herbal cigarette, in Queens Gardens. We were opposite the old cop-shop and in distant view of an actual cop. This was 'little old lady amusing' in itself as I'm now an ageing hippie. Then we went to the Hull

Wetherspoons for a drink and something to eat. My friend had said beforehand, "Look if you feel weird, don't worry, it will go away in ten minutes." I did suddenly start to feel very weird, and I was already wishing I hadn't inhaled so deeply. Everyone around me seemed odd and were behaving very strangely, like a dream sequence in a movie. I followed my friend downstairs to the loo and suddenly the giggles hit me as I remembered the 10-minutes thing. "Which ten minutes is that?" I asked my friend "The real 10 minutes or the 'stoner' 10 minutes: and how the hell do you measure the second one"? My friend was wrong. By any stretch of the concept of time, I was stoned for an hour or more and it seems two puffs of modern weed is one puff too many for a little old lady, especially one prone to paranoia. The home grown of my long distant youth and this new stinky stuff were clearly related in the same way as a Yorkshire terrier is related to a Rottweiler.

That being said, you certainly don't need to be stoned to feel distinctly spooked in a Hull 'Wethy's. '

The Flamenco dress

Reasons to be cheerful #2 I can now wear a flamenco dress! (down from size 20 before BC to 14 approx). No worries about the bag showing until after 4 kilometres of Romeria (procession). Then a little stop was required to smooth the line a bit.

Yesterday I had my 'revision' (as they call it here). My tests came out clear. Very happy of course. Next check up in 3 months.

Throat Problems

I went to the "Otorrinolaringologo" today. Try saying that with a mouthful of peas … or even without! Spanish for Ear nose and throat specialists. Apparently my throat is clear, and it is just chronic irritation possibly exaggerated by the Chemo. I've tried everything the pharmaceutical industry has to throw at it but now I know it's nothing "nasty" I can try alternative medicines and therapies. The "otorrino" suggested some nigella seed medicine and something to produce extra saliva.

Blood spot (FBC group)

> A question about stomas. Mine looks really neat, and I'm sure they've made a very good job of it but occasionally there's still a spot of blood always from the same place. Usually, if I'm cleaning glue from around the stoma. It also itches as it tries to heal in this place over and over. It's as if the hole in my skin is just a little small and so one side of the ileum is slightly pleated. Just asking if anyone else has this problem. Is it common?

This turned out to be an old stitch which eventually popped out.

Keeping it positive. What a sense of achievement I get from a full bag of 'blonde' wee AND a good night's sleep! RC and Urostomy is not such a bad result.

Sniffer Dogs?

No, I'm not back on the subject of cannabis!

I was just reminded about a report that suggested that dogs can smell cancer. I also remembered that in the couple of years leading up to my diagnosis, on and off, my urine would smell like chicken soup! I was confused about this at the time but found very few mentions of this phenomenon on the internet. It wasn't a horrible smell, just what you could call 'rich' and as I say, distinctly of chicken soup! Last year my Swiss friend's dogs wouldn't stop sniffing at my crotch. Maybe they are cancer sniffers! They could be extremely valuable if so! I must remember to tell her.

Bag or bucket (FBC group)

> Bag ladies & gents ... I was in Ikea the other day and saw a strange fold-up plastic bag thing. It's supposed to be a

cable holder. Ikea will hate this, but it's absolutely perfect for holding the night bag by your bed. It even has a slot through handle thing at the top which makes the perfect hole for your tube to slide through. Also, you can unfold it again to put it in your suitcase when travelling. It's not sealed up the sides, but you can put a bin liner in it. I've only once forgotten to put the valve in the correct position, and I could smell the wee when that happened. I'm thinking of stencilling "Gucci" on the side! Other people use a bucket, but I like my 'handbag'. I don't like the bed hangers and most people seem to agree you need a bucket or something to put the bag in.

Happy Christmas! (FBC group)

Happy Christmas everybody. For all the ladies staring at the possibility of having an RC with a stoma this next year. Reasons to be cheerful #4. Your Christmas onesie is much more comfortable at toilet time. No more trailing it and its hood on the floor or dropping the bobbles in the toilet pan just to go for a wee!

Valentines day joke

I hear it's been snowing rather a lot in parts of the UK. Watch out! The bladder cancer group ladies have been round with their 'plaggy bags' seeing if they can write their names. So if you see a woman's name written in the snow. Don't assume it's an over amorous Valentines day drunken guy, it may be a girlie celebrating a new ability!

Extension tubes (FBC group)

Does anyone not use their night bag extension tubes? Do you save them up? I could do with more as I only get one a month which seems unhygienic given that I can have a new bag every night. The tube is really heavily ridged and so it seems more difficult to ensure it's truly clean. Especially as I use well-water which isn't sterile. I can and do clean it, and I use an antiseptic liquid to finish, but would prefer to change a bit more often. Can pay postage and maybe swap something or just send a thank you. Or does anyone know where I can buy extra tubes?

I didn't have any luck with this appeal but I did learn to make my tube last a month by cleaning it out each day with Active Oxygen cleaner (sodium perchlorate). This was advised by my Pharmacist after he did some research. You don't need anything more expensive than that, and water which I mix at about 50/50, keep in a squeezy bottle and squirt into the extension tube. Then I rinse through with water and finally, rinse through with Spanish cologne from another squeezy bottle. You can make your own cologne by adding a little perfume or a couple of drops of essential oil to surgical alcohol and distilled water. I cut the extension tube in half as it's very long. In the morning when I'm disconnecting, I push one end of this tube into the other to form a ring until and then again after I clean it. I can have an overnight bag each night (on the co-pay system here) if I want, but I tend to rinse those out once or twice to cut down the amount of plastic I send to landfill.

Close the plug! (FBC Group)

Anyone else always forget to close the plug on their fresh urostomy bag? I used to, every time! I know, I know, I should take the whole bagful and put the plugs in all of them at once but I never do. I've learned now, and I do this only about once or twice a year. It still makes me feel very foolish, though!

I haven't mentioned waterproof mattress protectors. Of course these are a good idea. Our double bed is 2 narrow singles bolted together. I can have a protector but my husband doesn't need to.

Phantom bladder (FBC Group)

Sometimes the contents of my intestines/bowel sit on an old bladder nerve and convince me that I want a sit down wee! Frank said "Why not just respond to it by relaxing your muscles?" Of course he's right. Nothing happens.

Stomaversary (FBC group 31 Jan 2018)

It seems to have become a thing here, to announce your anniversaries. I rather like it and since I don't ever announce my birthdays (I might from now on, though) I'm going to announce my 'Stomaversary. ' Tomorrow 1st February my 'bag-for-life' will be one year old. Well, not actually the bag. My little raspberry has been with me in that position for exactly one year tomorrow!

In the mornings I wake up happy now. Disconnecting the extension tube and forming a ring of it then putting the lid on the night bag tube are like minor rituals of affirmation for me. I slept well and just as long as I liked because I never needed to get up and I am alive because of the 'op' which gave me my second bite of the cherry.

Missed Scan - FBC group

Absolutely gutted and annoyed with myself. I just missed my 3 month scan. How could I have forgotten to check the calendar? Especially as I have worrying twinges. AArgh! What have I done? It may take months to get another appointment!

One of the lovely FBC group members reminded me about my next one!

All clear - FBC group

I hardly like to say, when some of our friends are having a bad time at the moment (I think this might be called survivor guilt), I got another all clear for 3 more months yesterday. We have to count our wins!

Sending best wishes to all who are waiting for good news and fearing bad news. I had a little wobble because I still have the cough and then I got a bad stomach so I was worrying. I think we probably all do. I was surprised to get the good news, even though it's more usual for me to be positive!

'Transference'

Apparently it's pretty common to have a bit of a 'thing' for doctors and surgeons who have saved your life.

I had a strange crush on my second urologist. Even though he looks a little like a more attractive version of Mr Burns from the Simpsons. Maybe it's what they call 'transference' or more likely it is that once again I was happy to have found someone with whom I could have an intelligent conversation, and who didn't talk down to me.

My first urologist didn't give such a good impression at first meeting (though I've changed my mind about him since) when, having heard from me that I was making up a nutritional supplement, told me it wasn't a good idea "Because," he said, "Olives are fattening"! I had really expected the lecture on conventional versus alternative medicine but no, he was still in the 80s, hung up on oils being fattening. His team are actually right into cranberries, though they weren't my alternative of choice being rather acidic, and therefore irritating to my then bladder. I really wanted to point to my belly and ask him if he didn't think it was more likely that it was the enormous quantity of cake and biscuits, not to mention rather a lot of chocolate which had caused my weight gain. I decided that lecturing him on the Mediterranean diet, given his position and the fact that I clearly hadn't followed any of my own advice, was probably not such a good idea.

I've seen him around since, and he seems like a really nice guy. He was the great surgeon who gave me a surgery, free from bugs and very tidy indeed in all departments. 'Mr Oliver' we'll call him gets bonus points for that surgery, which in turn gets him absolute forgiveness for that 'daft' olives comment.

However I still rather like my 'Doctor Burns'; He's quietly spoken (though not that irritating 'too quiet'), and thoughtful. I found myself wanting to please him but I probably irritate him like I do most people in a position of power with my habit of wanting to know everything, and talking too much. When I saw his profile on FB I was once again 'smitten' by the fact he's a bit left leaning.

I hope I never have to see my 'weird-crush' again, though, because I hope the rest of my urinary system holds up for many years to come.

Walking

We went on the Camino de Santiago (a very famous pilgrim walk immortalised in the film "The Way") for 2 days last week. We walked 20 miles in 2 days. I know that's not an extraordinary amount but it was long enough to make our feet hurt. I have to say I loved it and want to go back and do the next stage as soon as possible. It was a great celebration of health just a year on from my surgery. I met a Korean with the largest blisters ever and gave him some Coloplast to stick on them. I think it might work, but obviously I don't know.

Mother's day thoughts - FBC group

> I was talking with my daughter yesterday about why BC seemed to be such a breeze for me when it's so hard for others, and I think for me it was this. Once I was in the system, I ceased to worry (at least almost completely) I could let those who were caring for me do their job. Previously in life I'd always had to be the strong one. As a single parent, particularly. Later I married my wonderful and very caring husband. Even after my kids had grown and gone though, I always had guilt about whether what I did as a mum was

enough. I handled much of the earning, the larger part of the DIY, etc. It was as though I was unable to let go. BC gave me the ability to be 'the patient'. The weak one rather than the strong. It was a revelation! I'm now back to being strong but with a different attitude. I now don't have to be a superwoman. I can say "I am enough." Not everyone has this I know but if you are struggling with the idea of not being the person you were ... let me tell you from my point of view. Relax. Let the surgeons do their work. Let your partner/family take the strain and be good to you and take time out from the guilt or the desire to be perfect. Afterwards, you can build a new better version of you. After letting go for a bit. Happy Mothers Day to the mothers and happy recovery to the dads and everyone else.

Data

It seems to me that nobody gets asked to feed back any statistical info to their medical team or anyone else before, during, or after their treatment. Info taken about my cancer and its possible causes (admittedly in Spain but I understand it's pretty much the same in the uk) So- Do you smoke No. Have you ever smoked? Yes, for 10 years but I gave up 30 years ago. Tick ... Smoking-related. The fact that I worked with plastics with chemical colourants all over my hands every day of the week seemed not to be important. That I had a sedentary lifestyle ... not important. My water-dodging ... seemingly not important ... Family history ... possible ... not noted ... Recent bereavement ... not noted ... Extremely stressful year or two causing changes in diet and behaviour ... nope not interested. They don't do any statistical analysis. Either before or after. I'm doing really well now (I hope) but are they interested in my new lifestyle or diet? Nahhhh! If I do well, my statistics will go down on the side of RC and Chemo but will show no link to other deliberate physical and psychological changes. We are missing SO much important data. Prevention, I'm afraid, isn't profitable.

Dramatic failure

I've often wondered what a spectacular bag failure would look like. Fortunately, when it happened I was in the toilet, just about to empty an overfull bag. I'd been editing videos (a new thing for me) and had got really into it and forgot. When I got there just the extra pressure of holding on to the bottom of the bag to try to pull the stopper out and the whole thing just flew off. Sploosh on the edge of the toilet seat and then 'flop' the bag rolled off and ended up on the floor. Weirdly the bag seemed to seal itself when upside down. I'm going to look at that by filling one up with water because I just don't know how that works! Well, I wouldn't like it to happen out and about. I've run off aeroplanes a couple of times and pushed past long queues of waiting ladies. I have always caught it in time. I have a feeling that this time the connecting ring wasn't well sealed as I was having difficulty hearing the 'click' the previous night. One more lesson learned!

I emptied it properly and popped it back on temporarily, but when I went down to change, I realised I'd then left the stopper out in my panic!

Nutritional medicine (FBC group Nov 2018)

> On the subject of 'nutritional medicine'. If we aren't allowed to discuss it, it will get pulled. I'm already on Lansoprazole for high stomach acid, but I've also had quite a lot of stomach pain which seems to flare up if I eat a lot of sugary stuff or have any alcohol. It could be anything of course, but it worries me because pancreatic and bladder cancer seem to have some relationship. Anyway, I've found a couple of things that seem to help. Homemade drinks containing fresh grated ginger (ginger carrot and turmeric is my fave but I also like celery apple and ginger) and a sachet of probiotics every now and then. I do read that ginger has other health benefits and I'm willing to go out on a limb and suggest that drinks like this might help with chemo nausea. Not expensive

anyway. So are we allowed to discuss our diets? I think we should, but not costly alternative miracle cures.

Leaks - FBC group

I had my first actual bag leak today. First in 2 years. I see messages from people having problems with leaking but apart from a couple of mistakes where I left the tap open, I've never had a problem. Until today! I thought people must be making mistakes. Now I know. Sometimes it just happens! Flippin' annoying but fortunately I was at home. I was teaching language one-to-one but fortunately my student knew my story so I could just beg her forgiveness, slip away and change. I'm finding I'm a bit matter-of-fact about stuff like this now, though. No point in getting embarrassed. Where would that get me? Easy to say I know. Much harder to cultivate a relaxed attitude, especially if you're working, or out in public.

I did have a leak in my night bag recently, three days in a row, which was very annoying as I thought it was me. It turned out that I had a dodgy set of bags. Maybe that explains why there hadn't been any supplies of that bag available for a few months. Fortunately, I'm a bit of a 'prepper' and so I had built up enough extra bags for 3 months and so I could just ride it out.

Gender confusion!

One of the oddest things that happened in the year or so after my op was that one day one of the little children in my babies' English class started staring at my neck and suddenly piped up (in Spanish), "Why have you got that on your neck? You only have one of those if you're a man!". I suddenly realised she was referring to Adam's apples. Well of course I haven't got one, but this little girl was convinced that I had (or had maybe confused bump with dip). Somewhat crazily I even checked that I hadn't developed one overnight! In any case I thought no more about it until months later when suddenly a few jigsaw pieces fell into place in my mind. When her mum had first signed her up she'd popped in while I was still in my PJs. I was a little embarrassed especially as my ostomy bag was in its night time sideways position, and that meant it hung down a bit sideways and a bit more visible than usual. It clicked. Oh dear. Maybe the silly woman did see me trying to hold my ostomy bag back. She may also have noted that I have started to wear a neck scarf more often because of my painful arthritic neck, maybe she put two and two together to make five and just maybe she'd been gossiping about it in front of her daughter about whether there just might be something a little unusual about me! I could have been very embarrassed but when I thought about it, it takes a very silly person to talk about things like that in front of a six year old anyway. I thought of confronting her ... for all of about 5 minutes, but remembered, you can't fix stupid.

Toilets

That story brings me to another point worth mentioning here. There was such a stupid epidemic of transphobia a few years ago that women with ostomies, especially in America where the stall doors seem to be higher, were contorting themselves into ridiculous positions in order to wee sitting down, so as not to appear to be standing to wee. Here is my twopenn'orth on the subject. For one thing it's much more comfortable to stand and if you can take one of the available benefits, you should! Of course if you find it's more comfortable for you to sit down or sit back to front or upside down (only joking) you do that. Here's another consideration though. Why should we allow peoples stupidity and narrow mindedness affect not only ourselves, but others too. We should literally stand against stupidity and in solidarity with our neighbours whatever their abilities, disabilities or even gender orientations are. If you kowtow to people who wilfully ignore that everyone has their story and their challenges then it's likely to come back to bite you in some way.

Also, while we're discussing toilets, I use the disabled toilet so I can wash my hands after handling toilet doors and immediately before handling the tap to my bag, and again after. If people want to look at me (apparently perfectly able bodied) sideways, I smile at them and say simply 'Ostomy'. Either they understand or they don't. That's not my problem. A friend gave me a key to the UK key scheme toilets. I think all ostomised people should have one as a matter of course. In fact I think all toilets should have sinks inside, but that's another matter.

Itchy skin (FBC group July 2019)

I've just posted this message on an ostomy support group but for members here who have an ostomy I think it's worth repeating:- There have often been questions on this group about itchy rashes under the attachment ring and I've often chipped in with the anti-fungal treatment. Well this week my rash has been really bad, and the itch has driven me crazy especially overnight. I then I remembered. I mostly gave up sugar to lose weight and because it's fairly widely believed that excess sugar causes inflammation and inflammation can add to the causes of cancer. Last week my friend bought me a load of food to take home from France. I say food, by weight more of it was sugar than anything. Having very little willpower I couldn't stop myself munching my way through far too much of it. Last night I realised that was what was causing my obvious fungal overgrowth! Doh! So, if you have massively itchy skin beneath your wafer it might be worth assessing how much sugar you eat. You might even lose a bit of weight as well if you cut it down.

Self worth (FBC group June 2019)

I'm an artist/craftsperson and teacher of crafts. When I went through cancer living in Spain I found it extraordinarily difficult because there was just no back up for me. I posted a few months ago how I'd got a fairly negative but typical response from some people, like, "you should have thought of that when you decided to be an artist" and about getting a proper job and saving for a pension. Anyway after feeling thoroughly slapped down by one comment I suddenly had absolutely the opposite reaction from the one the person who said 'it' expected me to have. I was terribly upset for a few days of course and then I woke myself up and said Hey. Why have I been teaching people to treat me this way through being apologetic for the job I do? I think often we get cancers at a low point in our lives when our immune system is low. I feel very strongly that a positive mental attitude has to be good for our recovery prospects and certainly can't do any harm. I'm now actually grateful to this person for the unwarranted slap. It woke me up! I now know how to value my work as well as myself. I was one of those artists who forgot my work was as valuable, and every one of my hours was as valuable as the next person's. We need to remind ourselves of that, whether we work or don't work.

I do think it's important to cultivate self-esteem and I have noticed that those who don't have it or don't develop it, struggle with getting through the changes cancer causes. Sometimes this means standing up against other people's judgements.

Exercise

There's nothing like having a 'bag for life' to show you how healthy a brisk walk is. I've noticed that if I have a reasonably long walk in the evenings my overnight bag gets fuller. Ipso facto walking helps your waste system. I believe your lymphatic system too. We're always being told stuff like this but I keep getting the proof! I just thought I'd remind you to walk the dog ... or if you haven't got a dog, walk the husband/wife. For your own health of course!

Another year (FBC 31 Dec 2019)

Happy new year to those who've made it through another year. Remembering those who haven't. Positivity is the best medicine. I'm convinced of it. So I'm raising a glass to life and keeping on thinking of all the best ways to live. If you have a terminal diagnosis, live as full and love as much as you can.

Zen and the art of ignoring sh** (2020, 3 years cancer Free)

This morning I woke from a dream. I have a very active and often very exciting dream life. In this dream I was visiting a friend, her husband and, for some reason, her husband's friend (a construct). I was couch-surfing and had overstayed my welcome. In my dreams I admit I still have some of my insecurities. In fact my dreams are where all my insecurities go to lick their wounds as I struggle to pretend that 'I'm so over it. ' You see, consciously I'm learning to let go, and it seems that, although it's taking a little longer, my unconscious is getting the idea too.

Since my brush with the reaper, I've consciously decided to try not to spend any more years winding myself up about other people's world view. Although it's taking some learning it worked! Whew! But this process is going to have to be repeated a few more times before my id gets it.

So in my dream my insecurity popped back up and said (out of the mouth of the friend of the friend) I'd been staying a bit too long. In my dream I stomped off in a strop and did the martyr bit on my own in the loo. Cue silly dream-invention of tightening my Fitbit, throwing away the packaging that for some reason I'd chosen to carry around with me on my (lone ???) hike.

My conscious decision not to give a sh** broke in, and told me to take a deep breath and just accept the situation. I woke up feeling on top of it, but pretty soon started going over long term family insecurities (which had obviously triggered the dream). A friend once told me "Kids make stuff up." Which is kind of shorthand for saying your family will always interpret situations according to their own world view. To be honest it's all of us. It would certainly be wonderful if we could all just learn that other people just plain see things differently and have the right to, and responsibility for, their own beliefs and actions. Obvious when you think about it, but how many of us still don't get it?

For now it's enough just to accept that I'm learning. Finally at the age of 60 ish I'm getting close to the zen art of 'ignoring sh**'!

3 years post BC and I managed to publish another book this week. My 3rd since RC! It's an open secret that it's me, but is a wee bit political. I know there are a few BC sufferers who've talked about writing that book. Just do it. You only live once. There IS life after RC. It can be an even better life. Especially if you can stop holding yourself back and stop apologising for being you.

Out walking

I just love Spanish kids. I also love linguistic differences. One evening we were walking down the road from our street down the long slow slope past the village name plate. We usually go past the bullring and the baby bullring, erected for the kids to play in, down to the big weighbridge where we would normally have a little kiss (another of our silly but sweet little rituals). Then we turn back for the long slow uphill stomp which would bring me some days depending on my level of fitness into the cardio zone on my fitness watch.

Often we would pass the group of girls, three of whom were my students. These girls seemed to have a cross between respect and a healthy enough teenage disrespect for me. Usually, though, they were very sweet as Spanish kids usually are towards their elders. That day, they decided to translate their greeting into English and I was the one giggling when, as we passed, they greeted me with "hello beautiful". How were they to know that no-one in England would dream of calling an old lady the equivalent of the ubiquitous "guapa" unless they were being very sarcastic indeed?!

Diuretic - 15 Aug 2020

Being a post-operative overnight drainage bag user has its upsides. I can see if I'm hydrated or dehydrated etc. by colour and quantity of urine. So, the last couple of nights my bag has been very full and very blonde. Anyway, I remembered I'd been eating a lot of raspberries and drinking raspberry infusion made from the 'pippy bits' separated from the dried powder I'd also made as a store cupboard basic. I had that sudden realisation. I'll bet raspberries are diuretic! I thought. So I looked it up.

"Raspberries are rich in vitamins, trace elements and secondary plant compounds and, as a result, they're said to have antibiotic, appetite-stimulating, diuretic and purgative properties. They also stimulate the body's defenses, support the immune system and boost metabolism."

My garden is producing 300 grams of raspberries every day right now, and that should carry on until maybe November here. Although the drying weather may last just a few more weeks. This is another one for my home 'can't do any harm within reasonable doses' medicine chest. If you could use a diuretic and aren't lucky enough to have a garden full of raspberries and a dry atmosphere to dry them in, I have seen raspberry powder at a reasonable price if you buy several tubs at a time. A little goes a long way. You have to look hard, though, because some of it is very expensive.

Swimming 'fun' - July 2021

Going to the swimming pool has been one of my greatest pleasures in the hot summers that we have where I live.

I worried that the water would lift my wafer, but it doesn't. I've no idea if it does for other brands but I find I can go my normal 5 plus days on the same ring both swimming and bathing. The very edge of the ring can go a bit whiter and separate for a couple of millimetres, but it doesn't detach at all. In fact, it never has. I swim almost every single day for 8 or 9 weeks in summer and it never has come off in 4 years (it's been 5 years since my operation but the pool was closed the first year of the Covid pandemic).

Since I've lost 25 kilos since before my cancer (deliberately) I can now get into a bikini! I prefer a boy-leg costume anyway, so I opt for the boy-leg shorts and that gives me more space for my 'tap' down the leg of the shorts. We don't go when there are lots of people so I'm not too worried these days even if people can see the outline of my wafer ring. I used to wear a pair of knickers under my costume to blur out the shape, but am much less self-conscious these days. After all, what would people be doing gazing at an old ladies belly to crotch region? And if they did, they'd either know … or they wouldn't. People aren't hung up on other people's appearance. We all need to recognise this fact I think. What a shame I didn't think that way more in my self-conscious years!

Unusual items in the bagging area (bulges in the crotch) are more of a problem, We don't stay at the pool long. Usually just 10 to 15 lengths and we're out and on our way back home so urine production is not usually a problem. Today, however, I realised that there was a little bulge rolled into my upper leg, I certainly don't want to have an obvious bulge, so I tried to make it even itself out a bit surreptitiously while showering off especially as there were some young girls walking in my direction. In the end I realised that any more 'fiddling' was just going to look weird, and maybe even creepy so I just flapped about a bit and shouted "can you find my towel?"' rather loudly at Frank. Not so much because I wanted him actually to find my towel, I knew exactly where it was, but more to divert any attention from the offending groin area. Rapid movement and loudness especially in a foreigner is just a little less embarrassing than packing a jumbo sized hot dog in one's pants … I always find.

Sex and relationships

Fortunately, our sex life was never the biggest part of our relationship. From day one even. We'd fallen in love without ever having laid a finger on each other and when sex did enter our lives I had been warned by my sister that the first time was likely to be a complete failure (she's very open on these subjects). She wasn't far from the truth to be honest. We simply 'got it out of the way'. Of course as our relationship grew so did our sex lives which became very happy, loving and just lightly experimental.

That was, until the time, a few years later when I thought my husband didn't appear to fancy me any more! I could tell that he still loved me and I was pretty sure there wasn't anyone else in his life, It was just that nothing was happening. At least not very often. Well It turned out that he had an undiagnosed illness and this was just a side effect. He got treated, and we quickly got back on track. We know now that we were lucky, we'd had this period and we weathered it. As my bladder cancer appeared I became less and less interested. Not only in penetrative sex which was frankly painful, but even in all the other things we could do ... used to do. My husband was incredibly patient and forgiving, and we always discussed it albeit sometimes for me a little tearfully. I did sometimes feel I was letting him down. Every now and then the interest level does bubble up to a point where we can play together again and when it does it comes on slowly and it can be very beautiful. Maybe I'm just a very lucky woman. I certainly think that my husband gets more love for his patience than he would if he were pushy! It must be harder for very young couples to weather this storm, though.

I was afraid of feeling ugly and freakish when I had my stoma and bag, but the RC for me was a lifesaving operation and my husband wants me around, so we've already come to terms with the bag and any little problems it might cause. We even welcome the notion because it means I have got through the other side of the operation and we'll have a chance of living another 20 years together. I can't deny I did have one wobble when my husband who had been taking refuge in Facebook accidentally sent the kissing fox icon to one of his FB friends who he'd actually met up with a few weeks earlier (he meant to post a wave which was a group 'thing'). It coincided with a very low point where it seemed my disease was terminal. I accused him of lining up girlfriends ready for after I was gone! I wonder if this is quite a common but unspoken fear. That we are replaceable.

I spoke about it with him immediately because I always do. I'm that kind of person. It's not always easy, but I tend to tell the truth even if it's unpalatable. If I hadn't voiced my concerns, one thing is for sure, even though it was nonsense, I would still be thinking it.

I personally think that voicing your fears and even letting the tears take over when they need to, helps. Even a tiny tantrum from time to time when things get too much helps you get back to normal quicker. It's no good expecting your partner to read your mind.

Well, we are now nearly 5 years into this new way of loving, and our relationship is stronger than ever. I'm sure my husband who is younger than me is missing out a bit but my self-esteem is so very strong now that I know he's lucky to have me and of course I'm very lucky to have him.

I do hear that, sadly, some relationships do break apart at the stress of cancer and the loss of sex drive or sexual attraction. Anyone who is suffering this loss on top of all the other potential losses cancer can cause needs to get some emotional support.

Ask your doctor to refer you, or ask your McMillan nurse to give advice.

You are not powerless

I don't believe that you are totally powerless when you have even the most devastating medical news. Of course some have an easier journey than others because of earlier diagnosis or stronger constitution both physically and mentally, but it's a journey and a partnership, or many partnerships. For all of us there are both medical and personal partnerships. You can't do it without your doctors, oncologists and surgeons as well as family and friends. Equally they can't do it without your input.

Someone who doesn't want to get better, won't get better. The best way to honour their work on your behalf and to honour the wonderful thing that is YOU is to do the very best you can to love yourself back to health both physically and mentally. Try and find all the help you need but also have some confidence in and respect for yourself. Listen to your body. Care for it. I don't necessarily believe in life after death, but I certainly believe in life before death and especially in my second life (the one that started when I realised that I only have one) can be the best life of all. For me cancer was a gift ... No, hear me out. For me, it was transformative. I changed my way of thinking entirely. I no longer fall into emotional traps that I used to fall into: because life is too short. I no longer undercharge for my work: because I now believe I have a value. I no longer say yes when I should say no: because I haven't time for all that. I no longer struggle with guilt and defensiveness (at least not for as long) because, in the end, most of the stuff that used to screw me up ... doesn't really matter. That's truly liberating!

The End

Of course none of us are destined to live forever. We can't ever know if our cancer will come back or if we will die of something else in the end. All we can do is stretch out the long tail of our lives as long as possible and enjoy every moment we have together with our loved ones.

I feel as if I'm less afraid of dying than most people I come across (while still having the 4am fears that I think everyone has). Partly this is because my Mum, who died and came back twice or three times in her life, told me stories of her experiences which lead me to have less fear. I think also partly I don't have a lot of 'unfinished business' either. I've had loads of fun and have left creative works behind me. I hope to have loads more time for fun and creativity. This might be an unpopular view, although I don't think there are very many great ways to die I do think having the opportunity to tell those people you care about how you feel before you go has to be something worth cherishing. I'm an atheist, and so I don't have the fear of judgement day. In any case I've only been the sort of naughty that only puritans would think of as naughty. I wouldn't want to spend an eternity with them anyway! A good few of my friends have left this life before me and I hope they have got the party well and truly started!

I wish you a successful journey wherever your illness or your loved one's illness takes you. Hopefully back to health with as few teething problems along the way as possible. I hope you find, in spite of the hard times, lots of humour, lots of positivity and lots of love and support.

Appendix

New Diagnosis? What to ask your Urologist

Make sure you take a list of possible questions to your medical team because it can be worrying coming away from a consultation having NOT asked the questions you want answered. Here is a list of possible questions to prompt you.

This list is NOT comprehensive and may have errors. It is only my understanding of the systems of evaluation. These may be different in other countries. I have put a dash between the letters and numbers. These would not normally appear on a doctor's evaluation.

What type of bladder cancer have I got?

What stage is my cancer?
(how far it has grown-'T 1-4') The higher the number the more advanced but even a T4 doesn't always mean a terminal diagnosis

How fast is it growing (grade)

Has the tumour invaded the bladder wall?

Are the lymph nodes affected
(N-0 means not, N-1 means they are affected)

Are there any signs of Metastasis?
(spreading to other organs - 'M-0 would mean not but M-1 would indicate that there has been spreading)

Some of these questions may not be answered by the first TURBT and a second operation may need to be performed to assess spread.

What are the possible treatments, and do I get a choice?

Which treatment do you recommend and why?

What are the benefits, drawbacks, risks and possible side effects of each treatment?

How will the treatment affect my day to day life/activities/work?

Will the treatment affect my sex life?

Ask your doctor for a printout of all your results and blood tests. They will always do that here in Spain. I'm not sure about the UK and US though.

If the doctor says something you don't understand, ask him/her to repeat it for clarification. Don't be afraid to say "What does that mean?". This saves both you and him/her

Join The Fight Bladder Cancer Facebook group

https://www. facebook.com/groups/124453424252307
They are very supportive and will point newbies at sources of information including their own website.

Thanks and acknowledgements

I'd like to thank all of my Patreon Patrons (Angie Scarr) for supporting me through the tough times in this book. My family both close and extended who helped me through. Some of them in completely unexpected ways. To my neighbours in my home village especially to Angeles, Montse and Inma. Of course to all the wonderful staff from Riotinto Hospital both those who are mentioned, and those not mentioned in these stories. Without you all I would not be here to tell the tales.

Thanks to all the members of Fight bladder cancer group. A special thank you to Melanie for generously given editing advice. I wasn't able to wait for more but I know that you would have helped me make further refinements!

To Rebekah from Livestrong and Rosie Mulley for nutritional advice.

I am always happy to hear from readers. Please do leave a review if you have found this information and these stories useful or reassuring.

For my other books do follow my profile on Amazon

I also write under the name Angie Scarr

search for: Making it Small - Angie Scarr

www.ingramcontent.com/pod-product-compliance
Lightning Source LLC
LaVergne TN
LVHW020429080526
838202LV00055B/5102